White Balloons

A MEMOIR

Jo St Claire

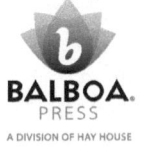

BALBOA.
PRESS
A DIVISION OF HAY HOUSE

Balboa Press books may be ordered through booksellers or by contacting:

Balboa Press
A Division of Hay House
1663 Liberty Drive
Bloomington, IN 47403
www.balboapress.com.au
1-(877) 407-4847

ISBN: 978-1-4525-0825-2 (sc)
ISBN: 978-1-4525-0828-3 (e)

Because of the dynamic nature of the Internet, any web addresses or links contained in this book may have changed since publication and may no longer be valid. The views expressed in this work are solely those of the author and do not necessarily reflect the views of the publisher, and the publisher hereby disclaims any responsibility for them.

The author of this book does not dispense medical advice or prescribe the use of any technique as a form of treatment for physical, emotional, or medical problems without the advice of a physician, either directly or indirectly. The intent of the author is only to offer information of a general nature to help you in your quest for emotional and spiritual well-being. In the event you use any of the information in this book for yourself, which is your constitutional right, the author and the publisher assume no responsibility for your actions.

Any people depicted in stock imagery provided by Thinkstock are models, and such images are being used for illustrative purposes only.
Certain stock imagery © Thinkstock.

Printed in the United States of America

Balboa Press rev. date: 11/30/2012

My journey through grief and search for inner peace—
physically, *emotionally*, and *spiritually*.

Contents

Acknowledgements...ix

Introduction xi

Chapter 1   The Day I Met Harley.......................................1

Chapter 2   In the Zone...7

Chapter 3   If Ever I Doubted..11

Chapter 4   White Balloons 15

Chapter 5   After Time 19

Chapter 6   First Christmas 27

Chapter 7   Roller-Coaster Ride 33

Chapter 8   Italy 39

Chapter 9   The Anniversary...47

Chapter 10 Love Is Love..51

Chapter 11 Permission...55

Chapter 12 Paradise 65

Chapter 13 On the Road Again..69

Chapter 14 Once upon a Time 79

Chapter 15 And All Your Walls 91

Chapter 16 Reflections..105

Endnote...109

Acknowledgements

I would like to sincerely thank the following people for the support they have given me during my journey with *White Balloons*, and in making my book a reality.

My *earth angels*: Gail, Kim, Penny, *Harley*, *Liz*, Gemma, Rowan, Kayla, members of LW Group, staff at Balboa Press, my beautiful family and friends; and all those who are part of my story.

Thank you also to my *heavenly angels* . . . my '*Spirit Guides*' . . . you know who you are . . .

'With deep gratitude',
Jo St. Claire

Introduction

We all deal with loss and grief in different ways depending on the circumstances. This is simply my story. The intention in sharing my journey is that others may identify with it and at the same time be helped and uplifted by the spiritual aspect of its telling.

The facts in this story are correct, as I know them; the thoughts are my own. I have written of events as they happened, but at times, I go back. I have changed the names of persons mentioned to protect their privacy. They gave me permission to do so.

I dedicate this book to all those who grieve.

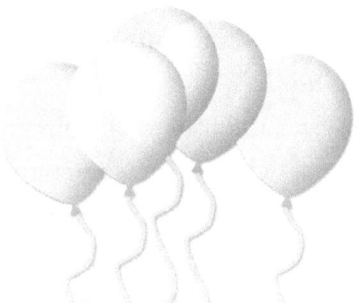

CHAPTER 1

The Day I Met Harley

(October-2009)

What a fine name, I thought as the fifty-something man in front of me introduced himself.

"I am Harley," he said. "I am a volunteer with palliative care."

I could not believe this was happening. My senses were reeling, and I felt that I was not in my body. I supposed that I needed to be removed from this unfolding drama, because physically and mentally, it was too much to cope with. I needed the strength to get through the time ahead and give my husband the support he needed.

I looked at my partner of forty-two years, who was lying in the white bed. It was him, but at the same time, it wasn't. Where had that man gone? He was so thin now, so weak, and his ashen face matched the sheets. A grey, stubbly beard had grown on his chin, but he did not want to shave; that would take too much effort, and he did not want me to remove it either.

He looked at me looking at him. "This is it, darl," he said softly. "I won't be coming home."

As he rested his eyes, the tears welled up in mine and tumbled down my face. That is when I felt something in my hand, and through my blurred vision, I saw a handkerchief there. I could tell straight away that this person, Harley, was a kindred soul; I could see in his eyes that he had suffered too.

My husband appeared to be sleeping now. He was exhausted by the events of the morning and the two-hour admission session. The palliative care team of his assigned doctor and nurses had been thorough in making him comfortable, cataloguing his history, and prescribing treatment.

Michael (Mike) had cancer of the prostate; he had been first diagnosed at fifty-one, and it had been a terrible shock. He had been treated with radiotherapy, and although there were side effects from this, he stayed in remission for the next ten years.

When the cancer returned, it came with a vengeance, and it had become very aggressive over the last year; he was now aged sixty-six. Recently, I had nursed him at home with the help of community nursing until it became too much for him and for me; he needed full-time care.

I sat down at the little table in the room, and the volunteer, Harley, sat opposite me. "This world is so unfair!" I exclaimed, and he agreed.

He told of a father he hadn't seen or spoken to in many years. That was until an amazing coincidence had occurred.

Harley had gone to an outdoor concert, along with thousands of others, to see Elton John perform. He was standing next to a man whom he recognised as a neighbour from a long time ago, a friend of his father.

The man told Harley that his father was seriously ill in hospital and not expected to live. Harley could not believe that this man was giving him a message, especially as his father had been on his mind lately. He had not wanted contact with his dad ever again, but now he felt a strong urge to see him.

Harley travelled to the place where his father lived and then found the hospital. When he entered the room, he saw his father, but the man's eyes were closed. Harley told me that he sat on a chair near the bed and looked on this man who had caused him so much grief. He did not try to rouse him; however, he was sure that his father knew that he was there, and then he left.

"The universe works in mysterious ways," Harley told me.

My heart went out to this man. I could tell he was a good person and had also been hurt by life.

"I agree," I said. "I have strong spiritual beliefs, and it has been quite a journey."

Harley was called away but said he would be back shortly. I sat quietly, thinking about the path I had been travelling for some time now.

I had been doing a lot of research over the last ten years or so. I had been looking for answers on how to establish a better way of living and how to overcome personal pain. It had been a mind-altering experience. I had read widely on spiritual matters and psychology. I discovered that the two went hand in hand.

Some years before my quest began in earnest, I had bought a copy of *The Power of Positive Thinking,* which was written by Norman Vincent Peale. I guess even at that time I had been reaching out for help. I had read it, but back then it did not resonate with me fully.

Later, I reread it and discovered many other books that aided me in changing my negative pattern of thinking. One of my favourites was *The Power of Now* by Eckhart Tolle.

It had taken a long time and much reinforcement to train my mind. Eventually, I was able to turn a dark thought into a lighter, more positive one. I had used this technique throughout Mike's illness. I told him that he could overcome this cancer. I was so sure! Sadly, he did not think about his condition in the same way.

Even when his doctor told us we could do no more to help him, I still had hope. But as I saw my husband decline, I had to concede that it was not to be. Then all I could do was reassure and comfort him with my knowledge through my faith that he would go on living and that I would be all right.

Along with training myself in positive thinking, I had searched for and found true belief in eternal life. As well as reading books, I had attended classes and workshops concerned with religion, mysticism, and meditation practises.

One of the classes I went to was called "Comparative Religions." At this stage in my learning, I was confused about religion. I did not know what I believed anymore. I had been brought up as a Roman Catholic, but as I grew older, I questioned some of the things that I had been taught.

I found the class's lessons interesting. The teacher and books covered the main religions: Buddhism, Hinduism, Islam, Christianity, and Judaism. I found that they all had a basic truth but at the same time different interpretations in their doctrines. I concluded that I did not want to be part of organised religion. I was glad of my Catholic upbringing—it had given me grounding—but at the same time, I felt that there was something missing.

There was a more mystical side that I hadn't learned about in Western philosophy but was part of Eastern religious teaching. However, what I was looking for was a personal relationship with God. I was searching for inner peace and looking for a guide.

Much of the literature that I read referred to the book titled *A Course in Miracles.* I promised myself that one day, I would read it, and eventually, I did. It was written by Helen Schucman, a psychologist, in collaboration with a colleague.

The book contained lessons based on spiritual principles and psychological thinking. The writer was said to be merely a scribe; the words came through the Holy Spirit. While Christian in content, it was not attached to any religious denomination.

I decided to do the twelve-month course, and this proved to be extremely challenging. The lessons I practised had a powerful effect on me. When I would do each one, I would feel a deep, relaxing peace; it was tangible and something that I had never felt before. The feeling would wear off, and I desperately wanted it to remain. I wanted this blissful state to be my constant way of being.

The lessons were not just about finding peace for oneself. They also contained exercises in sending that peace out to others in the world. They focused on love and forgiveness. This appealed to me because the work I was undertaking was not only for my benefit.

I had recently completed the learning, and I was now thinking differently; however, I still did not have complete peace of mind. The teachings said that the lessons would not bring immediate results. It was the beginning, but eventually, all would be accomplished. This was said to happen by a series of miracles.

I now realised that after my years of searching, Christ had always been the way for me. But my thinking had changed and broadened to include so much more. It was something that was now spiritual and not religious.

When Harley returned to the room, I asked if he had heard of the book called *A Course in Miracles*. He said that he hadn't, so I briefly described it to him and said that I had recently completed the course.

Looking then at my husband, I stopped talking. *This was not part of my plan!* I thought. *Who am I kidding? Am I deluded? Was all I believed in false? Had I brainwashed myself?* Mike was dying, and here I was talking about miracles . . . to a complete stranger!

I shrugged my shoulders, and turned away from the man opposite me. He, however, put his hand on my arm and gently said, "We do not know why these things happen, but from what you have told me, I would be interested in reading the book."

After I finished the book, I had a strong thought that I would not leave it on my shelf and that I would pass it on. Not only would I pass it on, but when the time came, I would also know who to give it to. I now knew that I was to give it to this man, so I told him that I would bring it in for him.

Harley smiled and said that he would not be back for two weeks; he only worked fortnightly on Mondays. I promised to leave it in the office next door for him just in case. He asked me to leave a note with my phone number so that he could return it later. I told him that wouldn't be necessary because when he had finished with it, he would know who to give it to.

I left the book for Harley, but I haven't seen him since. I wonder if he has read it, and if he is doing the "course."

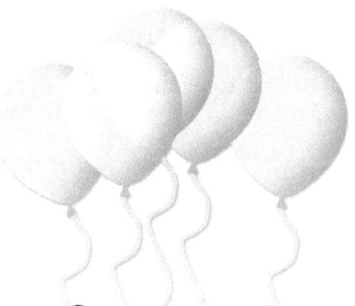

CHAPTER 2

In the Zone

As one day passed into another, nothing seemed real. Although I knew this time was coming, I was not prepared for the actuality of it, and I could not imagine how it was for my husband.

At first he was able to talk in between visits from the attending staff and his doctor; they made him as comfortable as possible and monitored his pain. I stayed with him, only returning home late at night. I asked if he wanted me to stay overnight, but he assured me that he was fine. I had been told that a bed could be brought into his special unit for me.

The doctor could not tell us how long it would be before the inevitable happened. He said that it would not happen in the next few days; it could be a week or two, but how many weeks he could not say.

I was coming from the car park on the day after Mike's admission when I met a young woman I knew. Anne was the daughter of friends from long ago, and we were both surprised to meet here.

"Have you someone in hospital?" I asked.

"Dad is in palliative care," she said. "He has leukaemia and hasn't long to live."

I was stunned at this news. Mike and Eddie, Anne's father, had been good friends when they had been younger. After Mike and I got together, we had spent some fun times with Eddie and his wife, Liz. In fact, they were godparents to our youngest daughter, Sheree, as we were to their youngest daughter, Marie. Sometime later, we moved away and lost contact, and sadly we had not seen each other for over thirty years.

Anne went on to say that her mother was staying at the hospital and that she would be pleased to see me. Eddie's room was just along the passage from Mike's. When I walked in and told Eddie and Liz why I was there, they, too, were as astounded as I was. We hugged and cried. There was so much to catch up on, and here we were, sharing the same experience.

This amazing coincidence brought with it much comfort in the time ahead; we did not feel so alone.

Eddie looked as bright as a button; it was hard to believe that his end would come at any time. He was still able to walk about, and he would visit Mike. Here were two old friends, both going on the same journey but now travelling the road together. This was comforting for both Liz and me, and more importantly, we hoped, for them.

Several days had passed, and Mike was deteriorating quickly now. One night, I told him that I did not want to leave him and asked if he wanted me to stay. He nodded his head. The staff soon arranged a bed for me in his room. This is where I wanted to be, close to my man, the man I had been with for so long. He needed me just as I needed him.

Whilst this time was extremely sad and very difficult to deal with, it was also quite spiritual. As I lay in the bed next to my husband, I pondered on what life was about. I had learned so much. It wasn't clear yet, but I felt great love and compassion for him like I never had before.

One night, I was awakened by the nurse entering the room. She had a different accent as she apologised for waking me, and her voice was soft and gentle. She checked on my husband and then sat on my bed. She said that she was originally from Sri Lanka. She was of tiny build, and she had very dark skin. Her eyes were so beautiful, and kindness shone through them. She told me that she had been on night duty since Mike's arrival.

"He is a special man," she said. They had talked about what was to come. Mike had told her of the love he had for his family, and he had said that he did not want to leave us. They had talked of the afterlife, sharing their beliefs. He told her that he had faith now and that it was all good.

She was to visit us again on the following nights. We may have been people from different backgrounds, but in spirit, we were the same.

Mike had not been a person of faith; he was a practical living man and could be quite negative in his thinking. He had little tolerance for introspection . . . or retrospection for that matter. He did not handle problems well, but then again, I guess, neither did I. However, throughout his suffering *I had to find new strength*, and armed with my burgeoning faith, I was now able to comfort him in a reassuring way.

I encouraged him with words of hope when we both knew that his time here was limited. I simply said, "Life goes on. This is not the end." I had learned so much over the past years, and this I knew to be true. For me, there was no question. I did not bombard him with my thinking because I knew that he needed to come to his own opinion. Instead, I did my best to uplift him, to see the light that was shining there.

Not long before entering hospital, Mike told me how much he loved me and appreciated all that I had done for him. These words were music to my ears. Our life together had been rocky at times; we had different personalities and often clashed, but the bond of true love was always there.

Mike, by his own admission, had been difficult to live with. He was unable to show his true feelings, but now he was loving and kind. And this was the way I had always wanted our lives together to be. This was a truly special time for us, a healing time. Sadly, in finding this, my husband was to die.

He told everyone who visited him now that it was "all good." This became his catch cry, and it was comforting for those who cared about him. Of course, he had times of distress and pain, but I was so thankful that the doctor and staff did all they could to make him comfortable. Because of this, he was more inwardly calm.

One day when the family was gathered around his bed, he heard one of our daughters comment on the fact that he looked really peaceful.

"I am in the zone," he said. "It is all good."

The medication had been increased, which accounted for his more relaxed state, but there was more to it. He talked of seeing his mother and father. His face was radiant, and when he spoke, there was such a blissful expression on his face.

"It is all good," he repeated. "I am in the zone."

It was easy for me to see that he was glimpsing heaven.

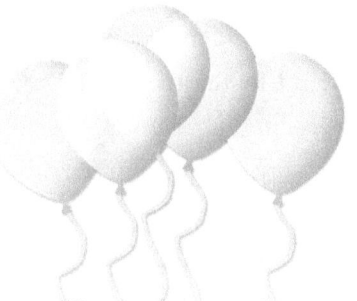

CHAPTER 3

If Ever I Doubted

The end time was approaching quickly now. Mike had been in palliative care for nearly two weeks, and his condition had worsened. The doctor and nurses were wonderful in attending to his needs. Medication had been increased to combat his pain and discomfort, but this sedated him more.

He roused sometimes and opened his eyes, but speaking was too difficult for him. Throughout this time, however, he was still lucid, and he rarely seemed disorientated. I would sit by his bed and hold his hand, and his lips would form the words, "I love you." I would tell him the same back.

Oh, what sweet sadness!

While Mike was sleeping, I would often wander the corridors. Sometimes I met Liz doing the same, and we would share the latest news on our husbands. We would embrace each other, and many a tear would fall.

At other times I would meet an "angel", like the hospital's resident social worker. I felt connected to her straight away. There was something deeply kind about her.

One day, I found myself outside her office, knocking on her door, and even though she appeared to be busy, she ushered me in. My emotions were overwhelming me. Mike was having a bad day, and his doctor had told me that he was fading quickly and that it could be any time now.

My anguished face would have said it all, and then a torrent of words fell out of my mouth. I talked for an hour or more with hardly a break. She listened quietly, but when there was a pause, she gently acknowledged my feelings. She knew only too well that I needed to release the huge load that my mind could no longer carry. Finally, it was done, and my words dried up. I wiped my eyes, and I felt lighter; it was almost like I was floating somewhere above this now.

While I had been at the hospital, I had often gone downstairs to a veranda that overlooked a beautiful garden. This part of the hospital was old. It had once been a fine home, and the garden reflected this. There were gorgeous shrubs, colourful flowers, and magnificent leafy trees reaching high into the sky. It was here I found solace; it was such a serene place to be. After my session with the social worker, I went there and just sat. I wanted to compose myself before I went back to Mike.

My gaze fell on a beautiful, weeping lilac tree. It had dew on its flowers, but to my mind, they were beads of tears. A tall green sycamore tree with long branches appeared to reach out to me. I leaned towards its leaves, and like a hand of delicate, lacy fingers, they gently brushed my face.

I was taking in the lovely scene in front of me when I saw a bright, double rainbow that arched right across the sky. I had never seen one like it before. It appeared in a luminous way. I felt a wave of peace and comfort pass through me as the words of the song "Somewhere over the Rainbow" came to me.

Feeling quite calm now, I went back upstairs. Our two daughters were there, and I saw their worried faces as they sat on each side of their father's bed. "Dad is going, isn't he?" one of them said. (It was more of a statement than a question.) "He is leaving us." Tears formed in their eyes as they held their father's hands and told him they loved him.

Louise, our eldest daughter, said that she needed to have some sleep. She had stayed at the hospital the previous night with me. We had slept very little because Mike's breathing had been laboured and he had been so restless. She lay down to have a nap but said, "Please wake me if anything looks like happening."

Sheree, our youngest daughter, still held her dad's hand. I had explained to both of them that when the time came, their father's breathing would slow down, and he may open his eyes before it stopped. Then he would be gone. I knew this from helping my father pass three years before.

Mike had been given the "sacrament of anointment for the sick and dying" by the hospital priest earlier in the day, and prayers had been said. It was very emotional. He had been given Holy Communion when he had first arrived in hospital, but he had declined the offer by the young African priest to hear his Confession. He had a grin on his face as he told him that there was not enough time left.

I left the chair by my husband's bed and was making a cup of tea when Sheree called me, "Mum, come quickly. Dad's breathing has slowed."

I rushed over and grabbed Mike's hand. His eyes opened, and he looked at us, as if to say, "It's time." And then he went. Sheree cried out in anguish to her sister asleep on the other bed, "Louise! Dad has gone!"

The rest of that day was a blur. Louise had been dreadfully upset that it had happened so quickly before we had had time to wake her, but I think her father was sparing her. He knew that she was not as emotionally strong as her sister. We sobbed and sobbed. It was so hard, but at the same time, we were relieved that our loved one's suffering was at an end and that his peace was seen so clearly on his face. Mike had gone. Only the shell of his body remained.

If ever I had doubted that we are spirit in this body, it was made plain to me. I saw it leave, and this truth was to come home so much more.

After all the formalities had been taken care of, we left the hospital. I had been dreading this moment of going back to a house that now would not feel like home. I had found this to be the case when Mike was in hospital, when I had to return to it at times. I had an empty feeling, and I felt so alone. I decided that there was no way that I could live there after he was gone.

As I entered the front door, I felt a wonderful sense of peace. *How strange*, I thought. *Why is it different now?* I was expressing this feeling to my daughters when the answer came to me. Of course! Hadn't I seen? Mike's spirit wasn't trapped in that sick body anymore. It was free, and he was here . . . with us!

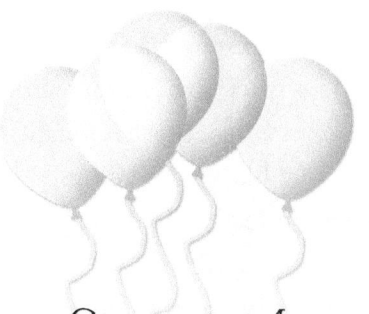

CHAPTER 4

White Balloons

It would take some time for the full, physical reality of losing my husband to set in. I had a deep ache in my heart that was so hard to bear. But there was so much to organise, and now lots of people were dropping by.

Mike had been a private man. He did not like a fuss. His wishes were for a small funeral with just family and close friends. I knew that he would like a simple service, not one that was particularly religious but one that was spiritual. I wanted it to be perfect for him.

We chose a celebrant we knew. She had officiated at our eldest daughter Louise's wedding. Patrick, a funeral director and the son of a friend, made the arrangements. He was extremely compassionate and kind. He asked for photographs of Mike to make a picture slide and for us to choose the music that we thought he would like to go with it. We chose "Little Old Wine Drinker Me" sung by Dean Martin. He was one of Mike's favourite singers.

I wrote the eulogy. I knew that he would not want me to ramble on, so I made it brief. But I included the parts that needed to be said. I wrote it in a way that I thought Mike would like. I did not make him sound like a saint because I knew that he would have no time for that. Instead, I tried to portray a man who loved his family and whom we loved back.

This was such an overwhelming time. Although we had been prepared for it, we were in shock. I do not think one can be fully ready for such a big loss. Nobody can know the true emotion of this until it happens. Of course, people are different, and not everybody feels the same. But if one truly loves that person, this event causes great pain.

Mike was well thought of by those who knew him, and now they showed how much they cared about us, his family, too. There were many beautiful flowers and cards sent, and friends came daily. This support was amazing. We would never have thought that so many felt sad at his passing, and now they were giving so much love to us.

It was a lovely spring day when his funeral was held, not a dark cloud in the sky. We, his family and friends, arrived at the chapel where the service was to be held. As the service began, we walked into the room behind the fine, polished wooden coffin with two dozen beautiful red roses on top. An updated version of "Somewhere over the Rainbow" and "What a Wonderful World" played, songs sung by Israel Kamakawiwo'ole. Our daughters had chosen the music for their dad. It was perfectly uplifting but at the same time sad.

I saw the gorgeous, white, helium-filled balloons sitting in a corner. I had wanted this simple touch as a symbol of peace. We wanted Mike to have that peace now, wherever he may be. There were enough balloons for each person there, and after the service, we would set them free.

The celebrant spoke on our behalf—emotionally and beautifully, she read a poem I had chosen called "Let Me Go" by an unknown author:

When I come to the end of the road
and the sun has set on me,
I want no rights in a gloom filled room,
why cry for a soul set free?
Miss me a little but not for long,
and not with your head bowed low.
Remember the love we once shared.
Miss me but let me go.
For this is a journey we all must take,
and each must go alone.
It's all part of a master's plan
a step on the road to home.
When you are lonely and sick of heart,
go to friends you know,
and bury your heads in doing good deeds.
Miss me but let me go!

These words I saw as true. I knew it would be difficult to let Mike go, but I also knew that he would always be with me. We left the chapel to the lovely song "Fields of Gold" by Sting, with each of us holding a white balloon on coloured string. We climbed up a grassy hill and gently let them go. They soon soared high into the sky, up, up into the clouds until they faded away, and it was done.

17

Sadly, the following day, I received a phone call from Liz, who said that Eddie had passed away just four days after Mike. Two friends from long ago had completed their journey; we felt sure that they were together somewhere.

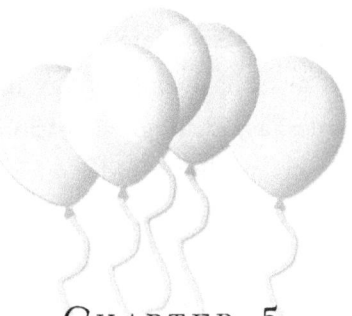

CHAPTER 5

After Time

The following days and weeks drifted into one another. I was exhausted and totally drained, and I missed Mike so much. For the first time in forty-two years, I was alone. I expected to see him come home, but of course, I knew he wouldn't. I had a small urn containing some of his ashes; the rest had been scattered at his favourite spot, where he wanted them to be. I planted a beautiful red rose and put the little urn underneath. I knew he would be pleased.

Emotionally, I was numb, and I really could not feel anything but emptiness inside. It was like part of me had died. Family came and went. My daughters did what they could to comfort me, but they were having a difficult time confronting life without their father and dealing with that loss. I thought at that time that I was unable to address their needs because my mind was detached, dealing with my own grief.

My friends were wonderful and did their best to understand. They did all they could to make this adjustment easier for me, and kindness came from everywhere. I was so grateful and full of love for them. I felt a strong loving energy through my physical body as well. At times, a soft, tingly sensation moved across my left shoulder and down my back, and I guessed it was the spirit of Mike comforting me. I had felt the same sensation, after my parents passed away.

I had talked of taking up writing for many years, but by the time I got around to it, my parents were old and ill. However, they encouraged me in this and told me that I could write a bestseller. It was after they passed(less than a month apart), and I was missing them, that I decided to write a family memoir. Every time I sat down at my computer, I felt this wonderful, peaceful feeling pass through me. I knew that Mum and Dad were happy that I was finally writing a story, and one that included them.

It took a little time for me to recognise that it was Mike with me now. I knew this instinctively. Whenever I was sad, he was there. I mentioned this to Liz, with whom I was developing a close bond because of what we had shared. I said to her, "I hope you don't think that I have gone mad!"

She assured me that she believed me and knew of others who had experienced this. She said, "You are lucky. I wish I felt that too."

I agreed with her but told her that while this was so comforting, I still had to go through the grieving process. I had to adjust to the physical separation and being on my own just as she did. As I mentioned earlier, I had been on a spiritual journey over the last ten years or so. This now held me in good stead, but I knew that I still had a way to go and obstacles to overcome before the path was clear.

Some years before, I went with my sister-in-law to a psychic expo. She was interested in numerology. While she was getting her "numbers" worked out, I wandered around. I came upon a woman who had gathered a large crowd. What I saw was fascinating! She was drawing in crayon, and what she was creating was truly amazing!

As I watched, a figure quickly appeared on the canvas. But from what I could see, it was not of this world. I heard her say to the person seated in front of her, "This is your spirit guide." Then she took the person aside, and I could hear no more. I decided then that I wanted her to do a drawing for me.

When my turn came around, I sat down, and the woman started to sketch. But it was as if she was merely holding the crayon and the "form" simply emerged. I was stunned!

Before me, I saw the beautiful, peaceful face of an Indian woman whose eyes emanated gentleness and compassion. Her face was all that could be seen. Her head was covered in a hooded garment, which was not distinct but made of swirling colours. They were mainly purple and mauve but edged with soft pink. The woman had written the name "Nyalli" on the right bottom corner of the paper.

At the top of Nyalli were birds, one on each side, and they faced outwardly left and right. I was told that they were eagles. Again, only their heads showed. The rest of them flowed down in the same colour. Between the eagles was a ball of golden light circled in red. From this orb ran a trail of white that entered Nyalli's head. It formed in a cloud on her forehead, and beneath was the circle of gold and red. The colours continued down and around where her body should have been. There, they gathered in the centre and appeared to spiral inward. The woman then spoke to me and told me what it all meant.

She said that she could see everything there to bring me complete peace of mind and happiness. Then she went on to say that Nyalli was one of my spirit guides (apparently, we have many) and that she had come to help me meditate, which would *assist* in bringing this new state of being about. The picture represented that which would happen eventually.

She then went on to say that the eagles had special meaning too. They were there to remind me that when this divine gift came through, I needed to accept it with wisdom and with grace. I was gobsmacked!

I took Nyalli home, and she helped me with the practise of meditation. I had found it difficult to meditate on past attempts. This was to be only one aspect of my spiritual journey. Back then, I had no idea of what lay ahead and how long it would take.

What this woman told me was confirmed by a New Age counsellor I consulted in later years. He read me the tarot cards that I had picked out, and they revealed much the same thing. But he told me there would be challenges to face first and deaths. Of course, this latter information startled me!

It was not long after this that my parents died; my father passed first and less than a month later, my mother went. One year after that, an uncle died. We had been close. He had been my confidant and my friend. Then Mike's cancer had returned, and he, too, was now gone.

Afterward, a woman from a community care service called to check up on me. I had taken up her offer of a session in grief counselling. She expressed the view that I had suffered "a lot of loss" in recent times. I certainly had to agree, but it wasn't just lately that I had experienced grief. I had been through deep, long-lasting grief before and a loss that had been extremely hard to bear.

It is amazing what an experienced counsellor can uncover. I didn't expect to be talking about something way in the past, but it just came out. The same thing happened when I talked to the social worker in palliative care and I knew that I was losing Mike. I wasn't thinking of that trauma from another time. It seemed to have no connection to the present situation. And besides, it was over. I had dealt with it. But it seemed it hadn't quite finished with me. I will tell you that story later on.

One day, I was feeling particularly tired and drained. I was sitting in my garden when a dragonfly passed by. I had not seen one since I was young, but now they had meaning for me. A dear friend had given me a lovely silver necklace for my sixtieth birthday, a dragonfly on a chain. I loved it and wore it most of the time. I looked up information online and found that the dragonfly was symbolic in a spiritual way.

It was said to concern the transference of illusion into truth, balance between heaven and earth, and life. There was much more written about it, but now as I saw this real dragonfly come so close to me, I realised that it was significant in a more personal way. It had been such an overwhelming time, and I had been doing far too much. It came to me that I needed to slow down and balance my days out.

Not long after this a friend of the family gave me a beautifully sculpted dragonfly as a gift to put in my garden. I placed it near Mike's ashes and the red rose tree.

After this, I tried to get more rest. I needed to because Christmas was approaching, the most spiritual time of the year. I knew this one would be difficult, but then I did not realise how much so!

One day, Sheree, my daughter, phoned. She sounded very upset, but at the same time, she was amazed. "Mum!" she said, "Guess what just happened?"

"Tell me," I asked.

"Someone crashed into my car where I had it parked on the street!"

"Oh, no," I said. Her dad had given her his car when he could no longer drive.

"I am so upset. It is damaged quite a bit."

"Never mind," I replied. "It can be fixed."

"That is not the point," she said. "It was Dad's car, and he looked after it so well!"

She then went on to tell me that when she saw the damaged car, she cried and cried. I understood that her emotions were still raw. The car her father had given to her towards the end had meant so much more!

"I was sobbing my eyes out," she said, "when a friend came by." And then she suddenly said, "Look up in the sky. You will not believe this, Mum, but when I looked up, there in the sky was a white balloon. It wasn't floating. It was perfectly still. I stopped crying, and a strong thought came to me: *Everything is all right! It is all good!*"

I was *amazed* by what my daughter was telling me! And I knew that she was thinking like me, thinking of the white balloons released for Mike as a symbol of peace on his farewell day. Now it seemed he was showing us he was still around and looking out for his family by sending back one of those *white balloons*.

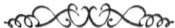

At times, I wasn't sure who I was anymore. I was completely overwhelmed. I felt that I was still married, and in my mind, I was; however, in the physical sense, I was on my own. It was like I had been transported back in time to a time when I was eighteen. I knew that I was sixty-one, but in a different way, I was that younger me before I had met Mike. It was so confusing, but somewhere in myself, I knew that it was part of the adjustment taking place.

In a way, it was exhilarating to be independent and free, but in another way, it was very lonely. I had mentioned this to well-meaning friends who were trying to understand the new me. "Don't worry," they said. "You won't be alone for long." While a little bit of me was flattered by this, any thought of someone else made me feel ill.

I was missing my companion of forty-two years. The nights were worse, and not having him to share meals with me was terrible. I knew from other widows that this was really difficult to get used to, but I did not want to replace him even if I could. I did not know what the future would bring and dismissed any thought of it. It was too painful yet. I could only live in the present, and from what I had learned, that was the only place to be.

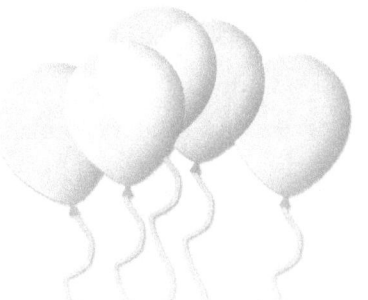

CHAPTER 6

First Christmas

I t was to be the first Christmas since knowing Mike that I would be without him. I didn't realise until writing this chapter and looking back that I had not known the true meaning of Christmas. I can see now that it is really profound, that the birth of Jesus that very first Christmas truly brought a saviour into the world.

Although it is commonly known that Christmas is the most difficult and emotionally challenging time after a person has lost a loved one, I was not fully prepared for this. The weeks preceding were busy, and I was still not clear in my thinking. It had only been two months since Mike had passed, and my mind was still consumed with what had been.

The festive season my family and I had planned was to be low-key. I tried to make an effort because I had always loved Christmas. I went to great strides to ensure Christmas Day was happy and fun, a real celebration of love. But Mike had been different to me. He couldn't understand all the fuss. When the time came, he enjoyed the company and party atmosphere, but the real meaning was lost on him.

Friends and others were so kind. They made a special effort to bring in Christmas for us this year. I could feel the emotion rising in me as it drew closer, and the week before, I could not control my feelings. They spilled out in a great outpouring of sadness and grief. But at the same time, there was an ever-present, wondrous love. This was to climax on Christmas Eve. Eventually, it would be fully shown.

It was two days before Christmas Day when I visited a woman whom I had come to know. I had gone to thank her for all she had done during Mike's passing. "I have something for you," she said. "It was given to me when my father died." She handed me a small piece of paper, and as I unfolded it, I saw that it was a poem.

"Please don't read it here. Take it home," she said.

I am so glad she said that because as I later read it—and you will see—the emotion it brought forth was almost too much to bear. Here is that Christmas poem by an unknown author (I have researched and been unable to find the original author.)

My First Christmas in Heaven

I see many Christmas trees on the earth below
with tiny lights reflecting in the snow.
The sight is so spectacular; please wipe away that tear,
for I am spending Christmas with Jesus Christ this year.
I hear the many Christmas songs that people hold so dear,
the sounds of music can't compare with the Christmas choir up here.
I have no words to tell you the joy their voices bring,
for it is beyond description to hear the angels sing.

I know how you must miss me; I see the pain inside your heart,
but I am not so far away, we are really not apart.
So be happy for me, dear ones, you know I hold you dear,
and be glad I am spending Christmas with Jesus Christ this year.
I send you each a special gift from my heavenly home above,
I send you each a memory of my undying love.
After all, love is the gift more precious than pure gold.
It was always most important in the stories Jesus told.
Please love and keep each other as our father said to do,
for I can't count the blessings of love he has for you.
So have a merry Christmas and wipe away the tear.
Remember I am spending Christmas with Jesus Christ.

Author unknown

The love and kindness shown to me that Christmas will never be forgotten. My heart opened wide as it all poured in.

It was the day before Christmas when the doorbell rang. I opened it to see four precious faces looking up at me. They belonged to the children who live next door. There are six children in the family. Sadly, another one had died when he was just a baby some years before. The parents had suffered much grief over losing the second child in their family. They had found it very difficult to overcome.

However, they had been blessed by five more, and along with the first born son, they had given them so much joy and love.

"Hello, what are you doing here?" I said, observing that the eldest was carrying a large parcel wrapped in Christmas paper.

"This is for you," he replied.

I showed great surprise as I ushered them inside, and I felt really overcome. I knew the family had a battle to make ends meet, and here were these gorgeous children, all dressed up for the occasion with a present for me.

When I opened it up, I couldn't believe my eyes. They had spent so much. Inside was a beautiful dressing gown, a lovely blue brooch with silver trim, pretty notepaper, and two recorded albums of Christmas carols.

I was completely blown away by this act of goodness and caring. I had often given them little things to help them along their way. And I had given them Christmas treats, but I didn't expect anything back. I could not help myself. I cried and cried.

Their parents knew what I was going through. They had suffered a huge loss. How hard it must have been for them that Christmas. They would not have expected to have one less gift under the Christmas tree.

Christmas Eve dawned bright and clear. I had never felt so emotionally filled in my life. I put my new Christmas albums on, and while I readied myself for the next day, I listened to the sweet, joyful sounds. When "Silent Night" played, it touched the depths of my heart and brought me to tears. I cried again and again.

I had been invited by friends of my daughter, Louise, to their place to join their family for a Christmas Eve celebration and to share special time in remembrance of recent loss. This family was suffering like us. They had lost a precious member to cancer. She had only been in her forties. I wasn't sure that I would be able to go. I thought it would be too sad, but afterward, I was so glad I did.

They made me very welcome as Christmas night came down. The adult's chat and laughter rang out as the children played around. I knew that they like me were wishing that their loved one was here. But we all did our best to be joyful at this truly holy time of the year.

I returned home to my simply decorated house. Sheree, my youngest daughter, called around, and I shared with her the poem "My First Christmas in Heaven." I read it out loud underneath a lamp outside. As the stars twinkled in the heavens, we knew that our loved one was truly aligned with all the majesty of the universe. He was surely spending Christmas with Jesus Christ.

It was quite late when I retired for the night, but it took me a while to go to sleep. I felt a strong energy within me that seemed to be part of my body. But I knew for certain who it was. It was not just any Christmas angel. It was Mike. He was letting me know he was with me in a very definite way, and I was sure he knew now what all the fuss was about.

The next day, Christmas Day, dawned magnificently. I had the family around, and the only child present was Sebastian, my youngest grandson. He was four years old and a real delight! Sadly, my other beautiful grandchildren couldn't be there. Kaitlyn worked for a shipping line. She was twenty (hard to believe), and William was eight and spending some time with his dad in Fiji.

We celebrated this day, which was especially put aside for that holy child so long ago. We tried to be happy and bright, but at times, it was difficult as we thought of our loved ones who were not here. At the end of the day, I received a lovely surprise. Another child was to be born sometime soon into our family. One member had gone, but another was on the way. This truly was a blessing.

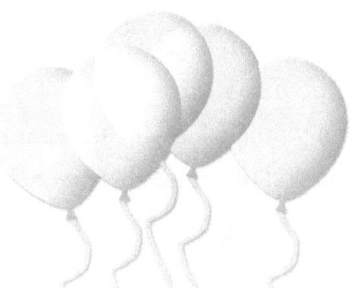

CHAPTER 7

Roller-Coaster Ride

The New Year came around, and I had been invited to spend it with family. On New Year's Eve, we went to a community celebration on a beautiful riverbank. The crowd gathered on the grass in happy celebration and great anticipation of bringing in another year. Like us, I am sure, they wanted this new year to be more peaceful and abundant than the one almost past.

There was plenty of entertainment for young and old, but for me, I was simply content being with my loved ones and taking in this colourful scene. The water with its silvery glow fed by the moon's gentle beams rippled softly in stark contrast to the noise and merriment it passed by. Up above, the stars sparkled delightedly in the clear night sky of the summer.

When midnight came, there were fireworks and mighty cheers as each embraced the other and invited in the New Year. I prayed that this one would bring all I had been wishing for. As I gazed up at the sky, a single star entered my sight. It appeared huge and crystal, sparkling bright. A wave of soothing peace swept through me. While I knew that this year would not be easy, I felt that gradually all would be made right.

I also knew that it would take some time for my goal of complete peace to be achieved. And of course, there were still within me strong feelings of grief. My mind was still foggy. I had read somewhere that it is nature's way to be like this. A veil of protection is provided as a buffer for the shock and pain until the adjustment is made.

From my misty mind, I could not see the future clearly, and sometimes I could not see it at all. Without warning, a deep longing would hit me and grab my inner being, manifesting into something real, and an aching that I can only describe as a physical void. It was one such time when I went to bed, feeling particularly sad, and I had the dream. I was thinking of what lay ahead, but in truth, I could not see it.

There were goals in my life I still held, but at that moment, I did not know if I could achieve them or if I wanted to. I had only been peeping at the year ahead since Mike's death. And as for anything past this time, it could not enter my mind. I knew my family needed me to be strong and live on, and I wanted to for them. But I could not see how it could be. I opened my bedside drawer and took out a pad and pen.

I wrote down a list of things that I wanted to fulfil in the year ahead, and then I made a ten-year plan. I put the list away. I could somewhat see the things that I had listed for the coming year, but as for the next decade, it was impossible to comprehend. I cried out in despair.

"Mike! I want to be with you!" Then I fell asleep.

I dreamed that I was staying at a beachside resort with some of my friends when a car with Mike inside pulled up. As I approached his car, he wound the window down.

"What are you doing here?" I asked.

"I have come to take you home," he said.

"But I am not ready!" I exclaimed. "None of my friends' partners have come to take them home."

The next morning, I remembered this dream vividly and knew instinctively that it was a message meant for me. I believed that dreams could be prophetic, especially after someone had passed. I did not need to think too much to know who this was from. Mike had been testing me. He had heard me calling out. I realised then that I wasn't ready to join him and that I had more living to do.

I still could not think too much about the future, but I started to contemplate the immediate year. I wanted to go on a trip, one I had yearned to do for so long, and now it was something that I pondered. If I was to do it, I needed to get strong because I felt so run-down. I had wanted to go to Italy for ages now. It was a passion of mine.

Mike had encouraged me to do it when he realised that he wouldn't be able to go along. I had a particular desire to visit a place called Positano. It was on the Amalfi Coast. Some years before, I had read a love story set there, and it sounded so beautiful. It was built on steep cliffs overlooking the sea.

The day after my dream, I visited my doctor for a check-up. He suggested that I may benefit from doing weight-bearing exercises to increase my strength and energy.

He went on to say that it had been scientifically proven that even a little time spent doing this each week helps to renew muscle tissue as well as strengthen bones. This was particularly important to do as one aged. I had on-going problems with muscle weakness and nerve damage from injuries received in a car accident many years before.

I thought about what my doctor had said and phoned a fitness centre that I found specifically catered to my needs. I had an assessment by a physiotherapist, and a weight-bearing program was organised for me.

I chose to have personal training, and a delightful young man was my instructor. He was very knowledgeable about physical well-being and exercise. I attended the training every week and soon started to feel stronger.

During these early months of my loss, I kept myself busy. I arranged my trip to Italy, and my granddaughter, Kaitlyn, decided that she would like to accompany me. I was grateful for this as I didn't want to travel alone and thought it would be fun having her along.

I also made some changes to my house. I had a deck built. I had wanted one for a long time, but for the last few years, this had not been a priority. Now I could do it, and I knew that I would relish time spent there, soaking in the view of mountains and sky and enjoying being outside.

Despite setting myself goals, I still had that empty feeling. Without warning, loneliness and longing would overcome me, and I found this was more so at night. I missed Mike's company badly; I cannot say that I missed everything about our relationship, but I mourned the loss of my mate of so many years.

I particularly felt this at Easter, probably because it is a spiritually significant time. While family and friends did their best to comfort me, it could not stop the feelings I had inside. These were the times that I would phone Liz. She knew what I was talking about.

During these last months, I had withdrawn somewhat from how my life had been. In the past, I had faced many challenging times and gone through much pain. I had been heavily involved with my family, taking on their problems. I had run myself ragged helping them out and had had little time left for me.

A counsellor I had consulted during this period asked me what my work was. I told him that I was in community welfare, and he had responded, "Ah, another rescuer!" I was quite offended by this, but as time went on, I believed that maybe he was right.

I guess I had acted out of love but at the same time perhaps out of guilt and fear. These were learned feelings, the counsellor said, that came from parents or significant others in childhood. He went on to say that no one was to blame and that it had been that way for people since time had begun. "We are indoctrinated," he said, "to think in a certain manner, but that can be changed."

I knew my life needed balance, and now that need had been forced on me. I was exhausted from years of neglecting my own needs, some of which I had no control over. Sheree, my youngest daughter, made the comment one day, "You have been living in a bubble lately, Mum." She had noticed that I wasn't involving myself in family affairs as I had done.

No wonder, I thought, but I knew that she didn't understand. She was not me and did not know what I had to do to cope with my loss. I understood that my daughters were grieving in their own ways. And as much as I felt for them, I realised that for each of us, it was very personal.

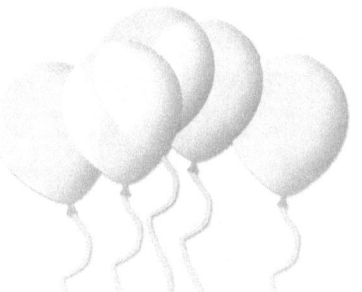

CHAPTER 8

Italy

(July-2010)

My holiday was approaching quickly now, and I looked forward to it with a mixture of excitement and slight apprehension. It would be a long flight from my home in Australia to Italy, and I had never travelled so far without Mike. He had been the one to take charge, and this had made me feel protected and safe. I would have my granddaughter with me, but I felt that I needed to be responsible for her.

Kaitlyn was a mature and independent young woman, but I was still her grandmother. At the same time, I knew that she would be a great help. She had a good sense of direction and a quick, young mind. I felt the trip would be beneficial for her as well. She missed her grandfather dearly. They had been very close. I knew he would want her to be there with me. I even wondered if he had something to do with the fact that she was coming along.

I received an e-mail from a younger cousin one day. I had told her of my wish to go to Italy and my desire to see the Amalfi Coast, particularly Positano. She said there was a shop she passed every morning on the way to her son's school. It was called "Positano," and she said it meant "embracing change and new things." She went on to say that maybe this applied to me now.

This was a coincidence. Some years before, I had bought a picture of a beautiful villa on steep cliffs overlooking the sea. It was not expensive, but I was strongly drawn to it. I had no idea where it was painted. There was tiny writing at the bottom of the canvas that I could not read, but I didn't bother to inspect it further.

Two or three years passed, and one day, I was dusting my bookshelf when a piece of paper fell out. It just had one word written on it, "Positano." It took some time before I remembered the story I had read many years ago. I must have written down the place where it was set. I suddenly remembered the picture, and after I grabbed a magnifying glass, I checked the inscription on the bottom. And sure enough, it was *Positano!*

I could not believe it. I felt strangely uplifted, almost euphoric. I felt that this trip to Italy was always meant to happen. I wondered how significant to my future it would be.

The day of our departure arrived, and I was very excited. I could only imagine what lay ahead. Our safety was not a concern because I knew Mike would be with us. This I had voiced to my daughters, thinking they may be anxious about our impending journey. They both surprised me by saying that they definitely agreed, that "he would be there!"

After a twenty-two-hour flight, we arrived at the busy Rome airport. It was very hot. Although we were tired, we were buoyed by the prospect of what lay ahead. We checked into our hotel, but we had no time to rest. We had to meet the tour director and the group of people we would be travelling with.

There were forty-three of us—twelve Australians, twenty-seven people from the United States, and a Canadian family of four. The group was made up of people of different ages ranging from fifteen to eighty years. I could hardly believe that I was here, and I felt that I needed to pinch myself. This had been my dream for so long, and I found it overwhelming.

Right from the start, Italy captured me. It took me straight to its heart. Even flying over it had been amazing. Its boot like shape, mountains, and pockets of green stirred in me a deep sense of something ancient.

In Rome, the sights were wondrous. There were buildings and monuments thousands of years old. I loved Vatican City, and St. Peter's Basilica was amazing, as was the Sistine Chapel. The magnificent artworks and Michelangelo's sculptures were divine. It was truly spiritual in every sense, and the chanting of monks in the background added to my state of bliss.

As we travelled throughout this beautiful country, I felt as if I was on a movie set. We saw the Leaning Tower of Pisa and then travelled to Florence, which was breathtakingly lovely. I was overawed at seeing the real statue of David. The Tuscan countryside was as I had imagined. Olive groves dotted the landscape, and gorgeous stone houses sat solidly on the land.

We visited a town called San Gimignano. It had been there since the fifteenth century, sitting high on a hill overlooking the picturesque countryside. One night, we dined at a lovely restaurant. I felt like Dianne Lane in the movie *Under the Tuscan Sun*, and I was so happy to be here. As we were serenaded by an Italian singer, I drank too much wine and danced.

We visited Milan and Lugano, a picture-perfect place just over the border in Switzerland, before we went to Lake Maggiore in Northern Italy. It had been a long day of travelling, and when we arrived at the Grande Dino Hotel, I felt completely overwhelmed.

The hotel was beautiful in an old-world way, and it was big with a grand entrance foyer. Giant chandeliers hung from the ceiling, and on its walls were magnificent paintings. The concierge was a fine-looking older woman, someone who looked like she had appeared from the past. When I entered our spacious room, I drew back the curtains, and my breath caught in my throat. I could not believe the beauty that was there. Before me was the most unbelievably gorgeous view I had ever seen. I burst into tears.

Before me was the stunning lake dotted with islands, and overlooking it were the Alps. In the late afternoon summer sun, the water shimmered brilliantly blue, and the sun's rays illuminated the mountain peaks. Palm trees edged the perfect lawn where it met the water along the hotel ground. *I must be in heaven*, I thought, and then I felt that strong energy pulsate through my body. It was natural to me now, and I knew it was Mike.

As I have mentioned, I experienced his presence many times since his passing. I knew he would be with Kaitlyn and me, looking after us as he had been at home. "You have arranged this," I sobbed out loud. I felt that he had helped me to achieve my dream of being in Italy. I was sure that he was working with God to bring joy for his family.

Looking back over the year, I could see some amazing changes in our family life. There had been lots of problems in the past, but now it was as if all this was fading away.

The next day, we travelled to a small island on Lake Maggiore called Isola Bella. As we approached the island, we could see a magnificent castle and glorious gardens surrounding it. We were taken by a guide through the castle, and afterwards, we were free to wander around.

This awesome place belonged to a family who had owned it for generations, and many famous people had stayed there—politicians, noblemen, including in later times, Prince Charles and Lady Diana. We were only shown part of the castle because much of it was the private residence of the present family.

The gardens were the loveliest I had ever seen. Like the rest of Italy, there were wonderful statues, such as that of Neptune and other iconic figures. They were placed among the brilliant flowering shrubs, garden beds, and the castle ramparts. Elegant white peacocks strutted around, pausing, happy to have their photos taken by admiring fans.

Our trip continued. We visited Venice, and again, I was overwhelmed at seeing this special place. I jumped about in joy when we had the good fortune to strike a flooded St. Mark's Square and had to wade through ankle-deep water to get to our hotel.

Later, we took a gondola ride and were blessed to have a tenor on board with accompanist on piano accordion. As we drifted through the canals of this beautiful old city to the heavenly strains of the music, I was lifted once more to that place of eternal bliss.

We spent the evening strolling around the maze of streets, and as darkness descended, we stood on top of the Rialto Bridge, watching Venice glide by. We wandered back to our hotel, tasting the smooth deliciousness of yet another gelato, its tangy flavour adding wonder in another sense.

The next day, we took a boat ride to Burano Island. We were greeted by brightly painted fishing boats bobbing merrily on a pretty blue Adriatic Sea. We walked along streets lined with pastel-coloured buildings and shopped, buying handmade lace gifts and other lovely things. At a local restaurant, we had an amazing six-course lunch of Italy's finest food and wine. In the late afternoon sun, we wandered back to the dock, fully sated with all this delightful place had to offer.

After we left Venice, we headed south to Assisi. The hotel we stayed at had the most magnificent view over the valley below. This place was spiritually driven with the focus on St. Francis. This was where he had been born, lived, and died. His tomb was located in the church named after him, and it was close to our hotel.

Then we travelled past the city of Naples and around the beautiful but steep Amalfi Coast to Sorrento. Kaitlyn and I were leaving the main group. We were having an extended stay in this part of Italy. We were sad to part from our lovely travelling companions, especially the ones we had become close to; however, we promised to keep in touch.

Two couples were staying on with us, and we looked forward to spending extra time with them. One pair was on their honeymoon, and the other was a married couple around my age. We visited the Isle of Capri, and its beauty lived up to what I had imagined. We were shown where scenes from the movie *It Started in Naples* were filmed, the film starring a young Sophia Loren.

When we went to Positano, I felt that it was every bit as wonderful as I had hoped. We visited this delightful place again before we left. It was beautiful and bright, sitting like a jewel, cascading down to the sea. It spoke to me of good life, the way it could be, not something transient but solid like the rock it was built on. It had been like this for so long.

We spent many hours browsing through the gorgeous little shops, taking photos of the villas suspended so perfectly there and the colourful beach scene. This was a place of fun and full of those who were seeking happy times.

Bright orange sun umbrellas dotted the beach, and the sea sparkled as holiday-makers in gay costumes frolicked along its shore. The sand was grey and coarse, but it was overlooked by the beauty and colour everywhere.

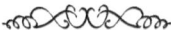

Later, I would reflect on my time there and what it meant for me. I came to the conclusion that it was about being happy and truly carefree. Maybe that was something that I could now embrace and live my life accordingly.

CHAPTER 9

The Anniversary

The holiday was over. I felt quite flat, and I missed Mike even more. To come home to an empty house after I had enjoyed the company of such great people and having had lots of fun was very hard to take. I had lots of wonderful memories and moments to share with my family and friends, but that could only suffice me for so long. The anniversary of my husband's passing was approaching. We decided to have a quiet family get-together to remember him.

In the days leading up to the date, I looked back to that time twelve months before. I felt sad when I remembered how it had been. It was hard to separate my thoughts and feelings. However, I made a conscious effort to think in the present time. It was clear to me. That was then, and this was now. But it did not stop the hurt and emptiness I still felt.

It was early spring, and the weather could be unpredictable. But on the day of the Anniversary, the sun shone warmly on our family as we enjoyed lunch outside in the garden. Later in the afternoon, we released helium-filled balloons. We watched them float up into the sky. These balloons were of bright colours. They were meant to be a symbol of happiness and freedom for our loved one.

I had talked to my daughters about feeling their father's presence over the last year. They had experienced their "own moments" with their dad. On the anniversary, I spoke of the need to let him go now. When we released the balloons, I sang out, "Go, Mike. Be happy and free!" Part of me didn't want this to happen and tore at my heart.

Sheree, always insightful, sensed my anguish and perhaps her own. She said, "Maybe Dad isn't ready yet and will go when he wants."

I had to agree because I didn't know what his agenda was He may have had unfinished business here. Perhaps he had an agreement with God to stay a little longer. Later that day, he visited me, and I wanted his comforting presence.

But as the days went on, I faced the stark reality that he was going. I could feel him fading and that this was final. He wasn't coming back. This impacted me in a very strong way. I had known this was going to happen; however, I had been distracted with my grief, and now it hit me with all its force! This was it. I was on my own now for the rest of my life.

This thinking made me feel depressed. I thought constantly of the time ahead. *How many years would I live for?* I was very grateful to have my beautiful family, wonderful friends, and my own interests, but there was a piece missing.

I knew to be whole and fulfilled, one needed to have all the parts in place. I was missing the love and companionship of my man. It was not perfect, but it had been there, hidden underneath that defensive shield Mike had around him.

Since his passing, I had still felt his love for me, and more directly than at any time during our marriage. He was free to show his feelings, I guessed. But I wished that *he* was still in this physical world with *me* and that *we* were as close *as we had been in the end.*

I knew that I would not actively seek anyone else. I also knew a relationship was something that would happen naturally if it was meant to be. I also considered the fact that I was getting older and was enjoying living alone. I did not need someone to live with me on an on-going basis. I was becoming independent in that way. I enjoyed my peace and quiet without having to attend to another's needs, but I was lonely. I detached myself from thinking about it and left it with God. I trusted that he knew what was best for me.

I was in transition, I knew, from what my life had been to one not yet determined. Days rolled into weeks, and at times, I still felt Mike with me but not as strongly as I had before. I knew he was gradually letting go. I was up and down in my moods, and sadness descended on me. This did not go unnoticed by my daughters, who both expressed grave concern for my well-being.

I could only be honest with them. I told them that I was going through change and another stage of the grieving process. Having always been open with them, I told them exactly how I was feeling. I told them that the reality had set in, and their father was leaving. He had to go now, and I felt so alone.

One morning, I awoke with a strong, urgent thought. I needed to do something to help me move on! It suddenly occurred to me that I needed to remove my wedding band from my finger. I was no longer married. In a symbolic way, this was keeping me joined to my husband, who had passed away. I knew instinctively that this would give me a sense of release and help the healing process.

It did not come off easily because it had been welded there for so long. But in desperation, I finally managed to separate it from my finger. Instantly, I felt a sense of relief and a feeling of freedom. I kept my engagement ring on as a symbol of our love, along with my mother's eternity ring.

I also put away a wedding photograph. I had had it blown up to a large size after Mike's death. I had placed it on a ledge facing my bed. While it had brought me much comfort in the past year, I no longer wanted it there. I kept small photos of him amongst other photos of loved ones.

Afterwards, I talked with my daughter Sheree and told her what I had done. She completely understood. She agreed that it would help me. She is spiritually free herself, and she had always maintained that she would never marry or have a wedding band. She thinks of it as a form of bondage and in some cases, a form of control, as in "you are mine now!" As she believes (and I had come to see), one doesn't need a piece of paper or a wedding ring to be committed to a relationship.

Sheree went on to tell me of her son William's Indian grandmother in Fiji, who had lost her husband some years ago. She said after a time, she had an "un-marrying" ceremony, as is done in Hindu culture. I could now see that in my own way, I had unmarried myself. Mike could go now in full peace. I had let him go. He could be completely free, and I hoped to be too.

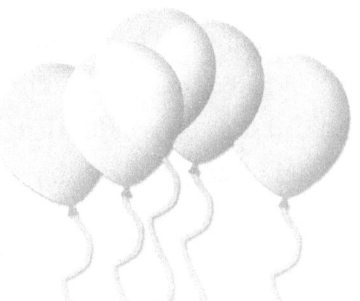

CHAPTER 10

Love Is Love

I stepped outside to have a break from my thoughts and my writing. I was greeted by absolute beauty. It was late spring, the best time of year, and I looked at my lovely garden.

When I returned from Italy, I created a little touch of its "soul" on my deck—a reminder to me of the wonder I had felt there and the glorious things that I had seen. I bought a statue of an angel with a large sunflower on her side. Her hands were crossed over her heart, and she had a lovely face; I named her Florence. Somehow, she comforted me and reminded me to have compassion for others.

I also purchased a lemon tree that I put in a gorgeous teal pot. I am delighted today to see it has flowered; its blossom is exquisite, and it smells so sweet. It has always reminded me of Sorrento, and the pot's colour has reminded me of the sea around Capri. A terracotta tub filled with fragrant herbs now sits alongside the tree.

I brought back from Italy two lovely tiles that show scenes of Positano and Sorrento. I glued them to a wall. On the railing, I put bright geraniums as I had seen on window ledges there. It gave me great pleasure to sit outside, simply observing all that is around me and remembering special times.

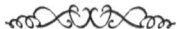

When my grief was new during that first year, I could not see the future. I felt such pain, but I decided that I needed to be around for my beautiful family. They would be devastated to lose me too, not that I would ever have contemplated ending my life. But I had known those who had followed their partners not long after and died of broken hearts.

Now over twelve months later and after a lot of soul-searching, I realised that it wasn't just my family I wanted to live for. I wanted to live for me! I have come to see that "love is . . . love" and that it is what it is. I believe that nothing can change or remove love. It will always be. True love is part of us. *We are connected to it . . . like a wave to the sea.* I believe that romantic love can fade, but I don't believe people can "fall out of real love." How can we?

At the same time, I know that love has no limit, no boundaries, and our divine heart is the size of the universe. We love different people in different ways, but at our core, it is all the same. But to be truly happy in a relationship with a partner in this physical world, one needs compatibility.

If another has gone physically, then doesn't it follow that we have to let them go mentally? I see people around me that get stuck. They think love is confined to a certain person. They cannot let go. To me, that is an obsessive love, a dependency, and a controlling bond. This applies if the person is still living on this planet or not.

Everyone is free! We just need to know that!

If a relationship is not complementary and it is beyond saving, what is the point of clinging to it? Someone said to me recently, "When my husband left me, my thought was that I wish he had died, because I lived in hope that he would come back. I really didn't want him back, but part of me clung to him."

Through no fault of our own, we can be dependent on another, but we don't often realise this. Or if we do, we do not know how to change the situation. This is when a professional counsellor can help, if one can take that step.

People need to fully connect to be completely happy in this world. Otherwise, we are only partly living. I believe that nobody needs to be alone and that one doesn't have to go searching. Simply free your mind and know what you want. Be open to it, and all will follow, if that is what your heart desires.

My darling daughter Louise came to visit me today, and I told her that I was starting the process of moving on. She listened carefully to what I had to say, and then she told me that she was glad because she had been so worried about me. I told her that it was not that I was looking for another man but that it would come if it was to be. It was more about me moving on personally as myself.

"Yes," she said. "You don't know what wonderful things lay ahead for you. Mum, and I am sure that you will get your writing published and have a literary career."

God bless her and all my dear family for having such faith in me.

It is still taking time, this moving on. I have seen that Rome wasn't built in a day. At this stage, I am mostly positive and bright, but I still have moments when I question what my life is about now. I have decided to go with the flow. It does take time to let go. However, I keep thinking of Mike's last words: "It is all good." And in my heart, I know that this is true.

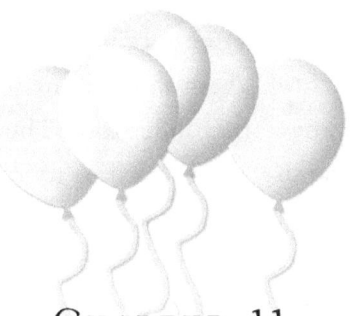

CHAPTER 11

Permission

Today, I visited a local mall, and I met a woman I knew from a time when we were children. We had been neighbours. I had seen her about from time to time over recent years, and sometimes we had brief chats. I knew that she had lost her husband. He had been killed in an accident nearly ten years before. While I had sympathised with her at the time, I hadn't really understood what she was going through. How could I?

On this occasion, I stopped and started to talk to her, and then I suggested that we might go for a coffee at a cafe nearby. Before we sat down, she introduced me to a man and a woman seated next to us. They suggested we join them because they knew each other well and often met here.

As the conversation flowed, it emerged that they belonged to a friendship group. They knew all about being alone. There were different reasons for it, but as they talked, there was a common theme. They talked of the different stages of grief that they had been through and the emotional turmoil.

They were at ease with one another and laughed a lot. I found myself relaxing too. I told them some of my story and about how I was still feeling. I knew they understood. They said that they met there every week and that I was welcome to join them at any time. They also suggested I go along to a group meeting. They said that they went out dancing and did other fun things too.

I appreciated their offer, but I declined. I told them that I thought it was great for anyone who wanted that. It was a different scene than what I was used to, and it felt alien to me. I knew there would be benefits to being part of such a group, but I also knew that most of those there would be looking for someone with whom they could be romantically linked. I did not want attention from any man I wasn't interested in. I didn't want endless dates in an attempt to find the right person.

I realised then that I wasn't ready for anything like that, and I wasn't sure that I ever would be. Later that day, I thought about being a single person now and compared it to how it was when I was married.

I could see that there had been certain expectations and obligations that I still mentally and emotionally carried with me. Forty-two years of being answerable to another had left a deep imprint on my psyche.

That is how it is when one promises to *love, honour, and obey*, but in reality, this vow can be misused and abused and result in one or the other feeling controlled. I can see how this happens when one partner has a stronger will than the other. And this was how it was with Mike and me. He wanted to have most of the say and all of my attention.

It was on my fiftieth birthday when I considered leaving our marriage. The day had started out very pleasantly. Mike had given me a lovely gift of a gold necklace and earrings. He was very pleased with himself and my reaction. He wasn't normally into giving presents. (I guessed our daughters had something to do with this.) But as the day went on, he became increasingly moody, and I couldn't understand why. *Perhaps it's because I'm receiving a lot of phone calls for my birthday*, I thought

A small party had been arranged for that night, with family members and close friends. Before the guests arrived, the tension between us had reached a boiling point! I was so upset, and I asked him what was wrong. He didn't reply and went off in a huff, but I had to pull myself together as the party was about to begin.

Somehow, I got through the night, but I felt that the others there would have seen my red eyes and sensed the tension between Mike and me. I put on the best face that I could, but my birthday had been ruined. I decided that I could not share our bed that night, and I would sleep in another room.

After the last guests left, I grabbed a nightgown and went there. Mike said nothing about this, but he didn't look pleased. As I entered the room, my gaze fell on a family portrait. It had been taken during a time that had not been particularly happy. In my present mood, it now added to my misery, so I took it down.

I put it in a cupboard, and as I did, I saw another picture, which I took out. This one was of Jesus Christ. It had been given to Sheree twelve months before by a friend from the Church of Latter-Day Saints. She had left it there when she stayed with us for a while. I thought about how beautiful it was and absent-mindedly placed it where the family portrait had hung in an alcove on the wall. I vaguely remembered Sheree saying that having a picture of Jesus displayed brought blessings.

I lay in bed, thinking about the day and puzzling over Mike's behaviour. Not that it was anything new, but I thought that he could have tried to be pleasant on this occasion. I guessed it was the usual reason. He liked to have all my attention and wanted me to have only his.

He had grown up like an only child. (His siblings were much older.) I had been told that he had been the centre of attention and wanted everything his own way. I guess that I didn't believe it back then. I felt at the end of my tether with his moodiness. Not that I was perfect, but I had tried my best to create harmony.

I was thinking these dark thoughts as I tossed and turned. Then my attention was diverted to the picture of Jesus. I thought once again about how lovely he looked, but his eyes were sad. I wasn't sure about religion anymore or what was true. *But there is no denying*, I thought, *you were a good man.*

My mind returned to my husband and what I was going to do. I was so tired of being unhappy. I decided that something had to change, or I would have to leave. I could see no alternative, but then I noticed that I was thinking quite clearly and formulating a plan.

I loved Mike, and I knew that he loved me. He was a "good man" in lots of ways. He had worked extremely hard to provide for his family, and he was reliable. He could not show his true feelings, and I wondered if this had something to do with the fact that he had spent four years in a Catholic boy's boarding school, only going home on school holidays. He told me that he had been not quite twelve when he had gone there, and he said that he had hated it, too.

I had read that this experience could have a detrimental effect on someone young, especially back then in the 1950s. They lived with and were educated by Catholic men called "brothers," and as he told me, the only women around were the housemaids. There had been little emotional support.

I weighed it all up, and the good in Mike outweighed the bad; however, I wanted us to be fully happy as a couple. I decided that I didn't want our marriage to end, and I would do all that I could to stop that from happening. I would talk with him about our relationship. I would tell him what I needed to be happy and ask him what he wanted from me.

After I came to this decision, I settled down. *Strange*, I thought, *how one moment my mind was in turmoil and then it has such clarity.* Before I had turned out the light, my glance fell on the picture of Jesus, *I wonder if you had something to do with this*, I mused.

The next evening when we settled down after a day of work, I broached the subject. I did the talking. Mike said nothing, but I tried to draw him out. It was like I was the counsellor and he was the client; however, it wasn't working. He wouldn't answer me. In the end, I retired to bed in the room where I had slept the night before. Oddly, I felt calm and was still thinking clearly. I knew that any change would take time, so I slept peacefully.

For the next two nights, I talked to Mike, but there was no response from him. Although he didn't say anything, he stayed put, and I hoped that he was taking in what I was saying. His face was impassive. Finally, I had said all that I could and went to bed in that other room.

This night, I couldn't settle. I felt frustrated at not making a breakthrough with Mike. *Or had I?* I asked myself. I wasn't sure.

It was later as I still lay thinking that I heard the crying, more like sobbing. Suddenly, a feeling of fear gripped my inner being. I could not tell where it was coming from. *Was it Mike?* I thought. I tiptoed to his room, and I did not let him see me as I peeked inside. He was lying back peacefully, reading a book.

Back in my room, I could still hear the sound of crying, and it was quite loud! I looked outside but could not hear it. By now, I was really afraid because the sound seemed to be inside the bedroom!

I looked at the picture, and I knew it had something to do with what I had heard! I quickly grabbed it and threw it in the cupboard and fled to the bed that I shared with Mike. He was asleep by then—or he pretended to be—and I felt instantly calm. This was where I was meant to be, I gathered!

The next morning, I woke late, and Mike had already left for work. I jumped out of bed, and there on the floor was a small red heart. It was made of a foil-like material. I had never seen it before, but it must have been around the house, I decided. I picked it up, and as I did, a strong thought came to me: *It is in your heart now.*

During the day, I was busy at my work, but when I had time, I reflected on the previous night. What had occurred had been extremely odd and something that I had never experienced before. And now I felt I was on such a high that I found it hard to concentrate. *What was it all about?* I wondered.

That night, Mike came home in a good mood, and he was talking for the first time in nearly a week. He didn't say anything specific. He hadn't had an epiphany, but he was smiling and happy. I guessed that he was pleased because I had returned to our bed. I couldn't tell him of how I had come to the bedroom. He wouldn't understand, and at that time, I didn't know what it meant!

What had occurred must have been of a spiritual nature, I presumed. What other explanation was there? I still felt high, which bordered on euphoria. But I couldn't explain it. After all, nothing had greatly been resolved . . . or not yet.

This state continued for the next two days. By then, I was feeling so tired and drained. In bed that night, I asked God to slow it down because it was too overwhelming for me. I couldn't function properly, being on such a continual high.

After that, I came down to a normal level of being and really began questioning what had happened. I worked with a young woman I knew had a leaning toward spiritual thinking. I told her briefly of my experience and asked if she had any ideas on what it could mean. She said that it sounded like what was written in the book *The Celestine Prophecy*. I hadn't heard of it.

She went on to say that the book was amazing and had sold millions of copies. When I told her about putting up the beautiful picture of Jesus, she said that related to that which was written in the "Fifth Insight" of the book.

"Through a mystical awareness and focus on "beauty" we can supply ourselves with nearly unlimited energy." (The Celestine Prophecy by James Redfield 1993)

She told me more but suggested that I might like to buy a copy.

I eventually did, and I found James Redfield's story to be a revelation. It was written as a tale, but throughout were messages with spiritual insights and psychology for living. I was interested in the chapter that dealt with "coincidences" of a meaningful type. The book said one needed to be alert to them because they happened all the time and led us on our quests for real answers to life.

I also mentioned my spiritual experience to Sheree, and she asked her Indian partner, a Hindu, what it could mean. He suggested that what I had heard on the night of my fiftieth birthday could have been Mike's spirit crying out to mine. According to his beliefs, when two spirits are joined together in true love and are separated, each will cry out for the other.

Although not a lot had changed with Mike's and my relationship, I was now on a personal path to find fulfilment. I realised that I couldn't change him but that I could learn about myself and the things that made us behave as we did. I hoped that by doing this, true harmony would come for us and within the family.

I started reading self-help books of every description, especially those written by psychologists. I would read a part at a time, reading sections over and over, underlining the words that I thought were particularly important and pertained to my situation. And at the same time, I read anything of a spiritual nature that appealed to my new way of thinking. The information I was seeking wasn't hard to find. Books literally fell into my hands.

Through this process, I learned a lot, and because I retained much of the information, I gained valuable insight into the human psyche as well as the real self.

Any relationship requires give and take, consideration of the other, and certain courtesies. Out of respect, one will seek the other's approval in considering certain personal plans. In a way, this is like asking permission to carry out a certain action. Then there is fidelity. I had always been faithful. I had taken my vows seriously. And although now it was no longer valid, I felt guilty if the thought of ever having another man crossed my mind.

It has taken time to realise that I do not have to think like this anymore. I have no one to answer to, only myself. I also saw that within my marriage, I had not been my true self. I had been mostly what was expected or what I thought I should be.

I see now that I need to give myself permission to live my life as I wish. I can choose what action to take and do the things that suit me. I no longer need to please anybody else with my decisions. I will always consider others' feelings, but for the first time in my life, I can be free.

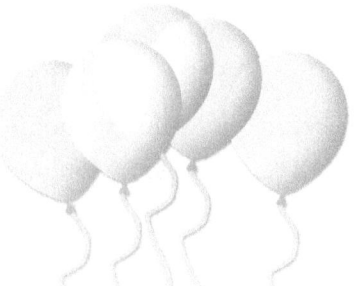

CHAPTER 12

Paradise

(2011)

The second Christmas without Mike had come and gone. I had been sad in the lead up to it but not as emotional as the previous year, and as the New Year came around, I knew that I was accepting his passing.

During a telephone conversation, Liz expressed the desire to visit Fiji. It was somewhere that I had wanted to go as well. I had often thought about going because my grandson, William, had been there to stay with his Indian father and family. I wanted to see this place where part of his cultural roots lay.

We planned to go in April, and after advice from a travel agent, we decided to visit the main island of Viti Levu but stay most of the time on an island in the Mammanuca group called Mana. While I wanted to visit Lautoka, the town where William's family lived, Liz and I agreed that one of the smaller islands sounded like a wonderful place to relax.

We decided to have ten days away—one night in Nadi on arrival and eight nights on Mana island—and to spend most of the last day in Lautoka before we would fly home the next morning. We felt this amount of time would be long enough, especially on a small island. How wrong we were.

Excitement was building in us as we arrived at the airport in Fiji. It was very colourful, and we were greeted by a handful of musicians singing welcome songs. Our accommodations were comfortable, and we shared a late dinner outside in the tropical night air. The palm trees swayed gently above as we dined near the lovely pool and anticipated the time ahead.

The next morning, we were transported to the port of Denaru, where we boarded a boat that would take us to Mana. It was an exciting journey, especially passing by gorgeous, white sand-fringed islands. When we reached our chosen island, Mana, a small boat had to come out and get us. The one we were on could not reach the jetty because of steerage problems.

With a thump, we landed on the beach, and straight away, I felt the impact. It was as if I was meant to be here, and at first glance, I fell in love with this place. It was as if I was coming home.

We were greeted by serenading Fijian men welcoming us to their island. One man officially greeted us and then led us through a beautiful garden of palm trees, frangipani, hibiscus, and other exotic plantings to the information centre. The man wearing his colourful shirt and Sulu skirt laughed and made light-hearted banter with us.

Later, we were led to our *bure* in the gorgeous tropical grounds and told that if we needed anything, he was our man. The men who brought our luggage to the door all chanted, "*Bulla*," to us with big wide smiles. In fact, everyone who passed greeted us in the same way. We agreed there and then that we had certainly come to paradise.

In the days ahead, we were in total bliss. We adored frolicking in the beautiful aquamarine water of the sea, a reef ran around the island, and gorgeous, brightly coloured fish swam beneath us. One day, we tried snorkelling, but because we had never attempted it before, we almost drowned from laughing. We did get some great photos for family and friends. The powdery sand of the beaches was the best I have ever seen.

Liz and I spent hours lying back on chairs under the palm trees, simply drinking in the magnificent view. We could see other islands and brightly coloured boats on the sea. Alongside the jetty, cruise boats docked, and yachts were moored. I expressed the thought that this was heaven on earth. Never had I felt so relaxed, and this island was having a spiritual effect on me.

I was amazed at breakfast on our first morning when the man singing and playing guitar (there was music everywhere) began to sing "Somewhere over the Rainbow" and "What a Wonderful World." It sent shivers through me.

That same day after we had arrived, the man who had met us on arrival came to visit. He wanted to know if we needed any assistance. Liz and I were surprised to see him, but it felt good to have a male looking out for us. We received lots of care from the staff during our stay, both men and women. We lapped up the attention, and after what we had both been through, it was just what we needed.

These lovely Fijian people were the friendliest we had ever known. It was a resort island with numerous activities; however, we were content to just relax and explore this idyllic place.

We walked to the staff village, where the Fijians lived in a simple, traditional way. We were delighted to visit the small school, where we met the headmaster and gorgeous children. We had been informed that the school really needed financial aid because some of the students were housed in a shed. They also needed more equipment, and we were asked if we could bring it to the attention of community organisations back home.

We spent eight nights on the island, and when the time came to go back to Nadi, we were very sad. They said farewell with songs that touched our hearts, and somehow, I knew it was not *moce* (pronounced mo-they, meaning good-bye). I personally felt such affinity with this place and its people. To me, it represented what paradise must truly resemble. I had never felt such peace and love. I hoped to take that energy back home with me, and I knew I would return sometime.

On the last day in Fiji, we visited Lautoka, and we were shown around the place where William's family had lived for generations. My grandson was very pleased that I went there, and so was I.

While I was happy to come home to see my loved ones, my heart ached for what I had experienced on Mana. How I had felt there was the way I wanted to feel always. I felt like my real self, totally relaxed and free. I have faith that will happen along the way. After all "mana" means magic.

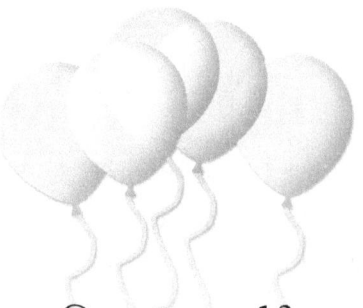

CHAPTER 13

On the Road Again

(May-2011)

It is eighteen months since Mike's passing, and I am almost healed. It has been a highly emotional and painful journey, but at the same time, it has been one of so many wonderful experiences. Most importantly, it has been a journey of love.

I have come to terms with the loss of Mike, but I haven't achieved complete inner peace . . . yet.

As I have mentioned before, this story has to a large degree, unfolded as it went along. I have gone back at times, and in parts, I have written of my own beliefs. That applies to this chapter as well. I am writing about events as they occur, but I'm including my own thoughts.

Although I have accepted Mike's passing and let him go, many amazing things are occurring. I feel that my memoir has wings of its own and that my story is turning into something bigger.

⸺⧓⧓⧓⸻

The first thing that I must mention is that I said Mike had gone. Well, I was wrong. He hasn't, not yet, not completely! I had been concerned that Mike may be trapped between heaven and earth as I had read of in stories, so I had asked him. I said, "Where are you, darling? Are you happy?"

A strong reply came into my mind: "I am in love!"

It took a moment after I had questioned this answer for another thought to come, one that said, "I am surrounded by it."

Then I trusted that he was indeed protected and reaching out from heaven. But I would be glad when he could forget about us and be fully at peace.

Yes, I did let him go, and I have. We are not attached like before, but it seems that he is still overseeing things. Perhaps he is making sure that the future he wants for his family is fully brought in. I feel him on my shoulder when I need a little comfort. And how do I know it is him now? I just do, and it has been proven to me.

About six months ago, I met up with a couple who had lived next door to Mike and me when our daughters were young. That was over thirty years ago. They had been friendly neighbours, and though we had lost touch, I had at times seen them around town.

On this occasion, we chatted for quite a while. They wanted to know how I was coping after I had lost Mike. I told them that it was not easy but that good things had been happening too and that I had just been to Italy. They were really interested to hear about my trip and invited me to visit. They asked me to bring my photos to show them.

I didn't find the time to go until recently, and it seemed strange to be there again, next door to where we had lived so long ago. When I entered the house, I felt the now familiar energy go across my left shoulder and my back. It was very intense, and suddenly, I realised who it was. Of course, it was Mike!

Another interesting coincidence occurred while I was there. I was given a gift from one that I had given them so many years before. It was a plant called a bromeliad. It had spiky, cactus like leaves, and I was told it produced lovely blue flowers. I could not recall giving the original plant to my neighbour.

She told me it produced offspring each year. She would pull the old plant out, and then she would put a new one in. Now she was giving me one of its pups to take home. It was hard to believe! I did some research and found out that bromeliads originated in South America and go back to ancient times, all the way to that of the Mayans and Incas. I guessed that there was some meaning attached to this. My old neighbour quoted me a verse from the Bible that says, "Cast your bread upon the waters, for you will find it after many days," (Ecclesiastes 11).

Not only after many days! I thought. *But in many ways!* To me, this plant is symbolic of that which has and is still happening.

(June 2011.) Now that I was clearer in my mind and on the road again, I looked at what else I wanted to achieve in my life. As I have mentioned before, I started to write stories after my parents passed away. It was something I had always had a yearning to do but didn't have the time. It was a form of therapy for me during the dark times and something that I really enjoyed.

I did not know if I had a talent for writing. My family really liked to read my stories and encouraged me. I did a course in creative writing, and that helped to develop my skills. I felt that I was "practising" for a few years—maybe for what was to come.

A series of "coincidences" have been occurring in recent times, leading me, it seems, to achieving my dreams.

Through my brother suffering a tragic illness, I have made a new friend. She and her husband have known him for a long time, and they have been very supportive of my brother as well as me.

She and I have connected in a spiritual way, just like in ways that are happening now with others I am meeting. In conversation, I told her that I enjoyed writing and that it was a great distraction for me. She told me that she had done a proofreading course and would like to read this story.

At that stage, it wasn't complete, and I was only half serious about doing anything with it. I had a vague thought that I may enter it in a competition of some sort. It was unedited, and I gave her a rough draft.

Several days later, she gave me feedback. This person was someone I trusted to give me an honest opinion, and being a new friend, she was removed from the essence of my story.

She said that she was totally amazed and that she thought that I was very talented. She went on to say that my story had made her cry but also that it had uplifted her and that she couldn't put it down.

I was overcome with emotion at hearing her words and hearing such positivity in her voice. I tried to remain humble, but I was excited now and thought that maybe I could achieve a lot more than I had realised when I had first set out.

I felt more confident now and looked at my writing in a new way. I earnestly considered the idea that I could possibly get published.

I had been thinking of late, *now that I am through with grieving, I need other interests in my life and other social outlets.* I had been doing a Pilates class for several months, which provided stimulating exercise for my body, but I needed to find more to occupy my mind.

I looked at what interest groups were available in my local area. I wasn't a dancer. I wasn't a singer or any of the things offered. Only writing seemed appealing. I discovered then that was what I was passionate about, so I knew a writing group would be perfect for me, especially now.

I had a membership to my state's writing organisation. People had recommended this when I had done the creative writing course some years before. I found that it kept me in touch with what was happening in the writing world. I had seen that there were a couple of groups in my hometown. Up until now, I hadn't thought of myself as a serious contender.

Now, however, I revisited this possibility, and although I still ventured with some trepidation, I joined one of the groups. I liked the woman's voice on the other end of the phone when I first took this step. She was welcoming and friendly. Later when I met her, we connected, and I felt comfortable being among people who had the same interest as me.

She has been writing for many years and has been successful in getting a lot of her work published. Already, she has been helpful to me. There are other authors in the group with similar success and some like myself. We are aiming to achieve individual goals. I am finding that being part of this group is giving me support with my writing, shared interest, and new friendships.

It was at the second meeting for me when I offered to have a piece of my story critiqued. I was told that it would be good if I could give the group an idea of what my book was about. I chose to give the title page, contents list, introduction, and first chapter. I was to e-mail this to the others before the next get-together. We met monthly.

Because of legal obligations with my chosen piece for critique, I needed to contact *Harley* (the man that I shared a conversation with in the first chapter of my story . . . the volunteer in palliative care at the hospital.) It was unusual how I was able to find him straight off. I wasn't sure if he would still be volunteering in palliative care. After all, it was by this time almost August, two years on.

I knew that the hospital wouldn't give out the information I wanted, so I looked in the phone book. There were a few surnames like his, but as we know most have only initials before their names. But there in big bold letters was his full Christian name, and I knew that it would be him.

I told him my name, and explained what I had called about. He took a little while to remember me, and then he was really surprised! He said that he would be delighted to assist me, and we arranged a time to meet up for coffee and a chat.

After the phone call, I thought about the twists and turns my life had taken since Mike's passing. And this had been another example . . . I found it astonishing that I would be meeting up with Harley again, and thinking of publishing a book!

I met with Harley this week, and what a delightful man he is—so compassionate and kind just as I remembered him. Again, I felt that spiritual connection. I was rather daunted when he told me of his credentials. I probably would not have met him if he had told me before. Then I would have had to abandon his part in my story.

What he told me when he sat down and started to read the few pages that I had brought with me really set me back. And afterwards, I was to be completely gobsmacked when I thought about it all!

Harley told me that he had done a lot of writing over the years. He then went on to say that he had a doctorate in management education and had completed a thesis of about 240,000 words!

I couldn't believe it! He went on reading the chapter, and then tears came to his eyes. He pulled a handkerchief out for himself this time.

He said he could really identify with what I had written and thought of his own mother when her time had come. He pointed out some typing errors to me and then said it was perfectly fine for me to use the part of my story concerning him.

In a very genuine way, Harley expressed how humble he felt that I had written about him. I said, that meeting him in palliative care, and the *conversation we had shared*, fitted in perfectly with my story. Then I asked if he had read the book that I had left for him, *A Course in Miracles*.

To my surprise, he was quite vague about this and couldn't seem to remember if he had gotten it. He asked me where I had left it, but he couldn't recall anything much about it. I told him that I had given it to a woman in the volunteer office next door to the room my husband had been in. I had left a note with his name and had asked the woman to leave it there for him.

I guess it was more part of my story than his—

I could see his mind ticking over, and then he said, "Maybe I can get a copy from the library." Or perhaps he will find the book is still there where I left it quite a while ago now. He is still volunteering at the same place. It will be interesting to find out.

I have a feeling that I will have further contact with Harley. When he finished reading the sample of my work, he expressed the desire to edit my story—that is, if I would let him. We will see what happens.

Who is humble now? I thought. I could not believe it! *The universe does certainly work in mysterious ways!*

(August 2011) I had another relative pass away this week. He was a much loved uncle of ninety. He and his wife of ninety-one still lived on their farm. I was called to stay with her just after it happened. He died peacefully at home. They had no children, and she had no blood relatives living here.

I wasn't looking forward to the sadness waiting there. While I thought of my uncle and happy times past, I wasn't mourning him. I felt great sympathy for his wife, but he had lived a good, long time. And because I knew absolutely that life went on after death, I did not shed a tear for him. I remembered him quietly and respectfully, especially when I wandered around the property where he had lived for so long. It was set among rolling paddocks, bushes, and hills. It was a perfect retreat.

My heart went out to his partner of sixty-six years. She would miss him terribly. However, I was able to tell her that I felt him there in the house and surrounding area. He hadn't left, and I told her that she would see him again, in the next life. I now had the same tingly sensation pass through me, and I felt his peace. Not only would she see him again, but so would I.

(September 2011) I received feedback from my writers' group this week regarding my piece for critique. I felt rather nervous about it beforehand, but I am very pleased with their comments. They all seemed to like my writing, using words like "fluid, punchy lines," "delightful, engaging style," and "easy to read." I was thrilled!

Of course, there were a few different opinions and suggestions. Some said that they couldn't find anything to change. But a couple of others selected parts that I may like to look at and gave me their ideas.

I took these opinions on board for consideration, and I have made amendments where I could see that they were warranted. After all, these comments were from experienced writers.

I now think that maybe I can get my story published, and I am certain that I will be guided.

"Dream lofty dreams and as you dream so shall you become. Your vision is the promise of what you shall one day be; your ideal is the prophecy of what you shall at last unveil." (This quote is from "As a Man Thinketh", by James Allen, 1864-1912.)

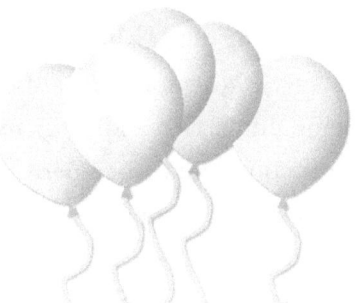

CHAPTER 14

Once upon a Time

This story, is one that I referred to in an earlier part of the book. (See—Chapter 5.) It happened a long time ago; however, it lived on in me for almost forty years. I was a young girl of seventeen when I was faced with no alternative but to give my baby away.

It was in the early 1960s when the unthinkable happened and I became pregnant. I had been going out with a boy for over a year. We were both the same age. For the first months, we were simply friends, and then nature had its way.

The contraceptive pill had just been released onto the market. But because I was a Roman Catholic and sex before marriage was considered a sin, there was no way that I would have gone to a doctor and asked for it. There were alternatives, but these methods were not reliable. Besides, we were so young, and we did not think of the consequences.

Marriage was discussed along with both our parents, but my boyfriend and I agreed that we weren't ready for that big step.

Back at that time, bringing up a child on one's own was not acceptable within society. No monetary assistance was given by the government. Being unmarried and pregnant was looked on as a sin. The woman was considered a bad person and thought of as promiscuous when most were simply naïve and innocent young women.

Choices were limited. My parents couldn't add another child to an already overburdened family. I didn't expect them to. In fact, it wasn't even discussed with me at the time. It was years later when my mother told me that she had wanted to help raise my baby but my father hadn't allowed it.

Actually, nothing really much had been said about the situation; it was so hush-hush! They only asked, "Do you want to get married?" and when I said no, they asked, "What do you want to do?"

I saw no option but to adopt my baby out. I thought it was best for the child I was carrying. I hadn't considered abortion because I was a Roman Catholic and it was not a legal practise back then. It was carried out secretly, but people knew it was highly dangerous.

I knew that there were couples who desperately wanted children, who could have none of their own. I wanted the child that I was carrying to have advantages in life.

When the time got close, I was whisked away to a home for unwed mothers-to-be. I didn't think too much about it then. I simply knew what I had to do. I remember that the labour was long and hard and that I felt so alone.

When my baby girl was born, I clasped her tight, but then I realised that she wasn't mine and that I had to give her away. That is when the full impact hit me, and with *great force*.

I felt so sad, but uppermost in my mind was the thought that I had to do it. There was no going back.

After the formalities were dealt with, I returned home. I felt numb like someone had ripped my heart out.

I had been told that once the papers were signed, there would be no going back. It was a totally binding, legal agreement. There was a cooling-off period before this was done, but I knew that there was no other way.

I tried to move on with my life, but I felt empty inside and believed that my future was ruined. To add to my misery, I felt like an outcast in my small hometown. Even though my parents did their best to keep things quiet, I could sense the covert looks and sly whispers. Secrets always have a way of escaping in places like that.

Many years later, I realised that I had not been prepared for the emotional effect of giving up my baby. I felt so guilty, and though I had done it with the best of intentions, it hurt me. I felt like a bad person, and I was deeply grieving my loss. There had been no counselling. I was expected to just get on with life.

I was too ashamed to talk to anyone about what had happened. I kept it to myself, and no one mentioned it. My mother tried to, and my father said nothing. I didn't blame my parents, and I still don't. This is how it was. I see now that they didn't know what to say.

Time went by. Somehow, I managed to get on with my life, and then I met Mike. He was a few years older than I was, and he was a steadying influence. After we had known each other for six months, he asked me to marry him, and this time, I agreed, because I knew that it was right.

Before I said yes, I told him what had happened sometime before I had met him. Although I hadn't spoken of it to anyone else, I felt that I owed him that much. He seemed to take it in his stride and asked very few questions. He said that it didn't make any difference. I guess he was as much in love with me as I was with him, and some months later, we were married.

While we were happy in those first years, a deep longing would at times come over me. I hadn't got over my loss, and I didn't know if I ever would. However, when our first daughter was born, I felt secure bringing her into the world. Less than two years later, our second daughter arrived, and our family was complete.

In those early years of my marriage, I was kept busy by raising our children and being a wife. This left little time to dwell on the past; however, it was still there, and it still hurt. I deliberately forgot the birthday of the child I had adopted out. It was simply too painful to remember.

Time passed, and our girls were growing up quickly. Now and again, I would think of that other child and wonder what she looked like. Over the years, I had often looked at young faces in the street and wondered if any of them were her. I didn't know where she lived, whether it was here or far away. I had no idea because I had been given no details.

I still had not told anyone about my secret, except Mike, and he never brought it up. At times I hinted at it when I was with my friends. But I felt too ashamed to come out and tell them everything and how it still felt. I kept this to myself.

It is well known that keeping painful emotions locked inside will sometimes evolve into severe depression and possibly result in a breakdown. In time, this nearly happened to me as I suffered worsening bouts of mind-crippling anxiety. (Years later, I was to read that relinquishing a child produced one of life's greatest traumas.)

Eventually, I decided that I had to talk to someone. Counselling wasn't something one sought out in those days. Firstly, there weren't really any counsellors around, and secondly, one would be thought of as mad. There were psychiatrists; however, most people were dragged off to them, and I certainly didn't want that to happen.

I spoke to our local priest. (I guess that I still felt like a sinner.) I was still going to church at this stage, and our daughters were being raised in the Catholic faith. They also attended a convent school nearby.

I told him that I needed to talk to him like I had at Confession. He was a kind man, and I had always found him easy to relate to. I knew that he would be compassionate, and although he wouldn't be able to fully understand the situation, being a priest and a man, I was sure he would bestow on me God's blessing and forgiveness.

He listened carefully to what I had to say and then quietly said, "You were young when this happened." He then went on to give me some prayers to say as an act of penance. He then blessed me in the name of "the Father, the Son, and the Holy Spirit."

After this, I did feel better and found that I could at last talk about it with those I wished to confide in. I told my daughters when I thought they were old enough. They asked no questions as I told them we would never be able to see her.

I put it away and thought it was gone forever, but then the laws regarding adoption changed. Access through legal channels was possible to allow for contact. If a party didn't want this, a veto had to be registered to stop it from happening. I thought about doing this, but something stopped me from carrying it out.

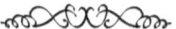

Many years later—in fact, almost ten years ago—a letter arrived that turned my world upside down! It just came out of the blue! There was no warning.

It was from a young woman who said that I was her birth mother and that she wanted to make contact. Of course, I was in shock! This was after thirty-six years!

I read it over and over and sobbed my heart out. I simply did not know what to do. I had buried it deep, but it had lain in waiting for this day.

After days of crying and considering the options, I decided that it was simply too difficult. I had my family to consider. My aged parents were ill, and I did not think that they would handle the news well. It could have been detrimental to their health. Then there were my daughters and husband. What would they think? We had not discussed it—only briefly in all those years.

I knew that it would have been an emotional upheaval in their lives and something that they may not have wanted. I talked to Mike about it, but he said very little, only that it was for me to decide. He seemed threatened by the news. I guessed that he felt threatened because this baby was something we had not shared.

I sent a letter back explaining my past actions, saying that I hoped that she had been happy in her adoptive family. But I also said that I could not see her. I thought that would be that and I would get on with my life.

However, once I knew her name and that she lived in the same small city as me, I could not forget. Once again, I found myself scanning the faces in the crowd and wondering.

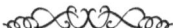

During the next two years, she was constantly on my mind, but I was kept busy with other issues. One day towards the end of the second year, I saw an article in the local newspaper that stunned me! There was a photo, and underneath was a name. The young woman was seated at a piano. I knew it was her instinctively. She looked so much like me.

I could not believe that I was seeing her for the first time since she was that tiny new-born baby! I studied the photo for hours. I finally cut it out and put it away.

Over the following weeks, I often got the photo out. I told myself if I could not meet her in this life, then I would in the next. My spiritual journey was underway, and I believed that emphatically.

But God must have had other ideas.

One night, the phone rang. My senses reeled as I heard the male voice on the other end say who was calling. I couldn't believe it after all those years! He apologised for disturbing me but said that he needed to talk to me about an important matter.

He said that a young woman had phoned him and said that he was her biological father. He said that he had been flabbergasted and wanted me to confirm that it was true. I quietly told him that she was indeed his daughter. Then he went on to say that she had asked him to phone me to find out why I couldn't meet her.

My mind was whirling. It was so overwhelming! I mumbled that I couldn't and hung up the phone.

The next day after a sleepless night, I finally decided that I *did* want to meet her in this life—come what may! And it seemed that she really wanted to meet me. I owed her that.

It took some time for this to come about, but I knew that there was no going back. I phoned a number that I found in the phone book and got an answering machine. When I heard her sweet voice for the first time, I almost cried, but I managed to leave a short message asking her to call me.

Eventually, she phoned me. She said that it had taken her a while to summon up the courage to call back. I could hardly believe that I was talking with her. We agreed to meet, but I told her that it would have to be somewhere discreet and that it would have to stay just between us for now.

I told Mike, but I didn't tell our daughters or my parents just yet. I didn't know how it would turn out. *We might not connect,* I thought. I had heard other stories of reunions. Not all had positive outcomes, and I did not want to upset my family unnecessarily.

The day arrived for us to meet, and I felt very nervous. I can't adequately describe in words how emotional and keyed up I was. I imagined that she would feel similarly.

When I saw her for the first time since she was a baby, it was surreal! I felt like I was acting out a scene from a movie, and I expected to see cameras recording every detail of our reunion. We hugged and cried, and straight away, I felt the connection. I knew then that we would have an on-going relationship.

I was so happy when she told me that she had a wonderful childhood with loving parents. Sadly, though, her mother had died when she was just nineteen. (She was now thirty-eight.) I wondered if this was part of her reason for contacting me.

It also emerged that she had been taught piano as a child and was now a music teacher. From what she had told me of her accomplishments, I gathered that she must have been very talented. She did not talk in a boasting way, but she simply talked about how it was.

She was a lovely young woman and seemed very mature. She said that she understood completely why I had given her up for adoption. Before we parted, we planned another meeting in two weeks' time. I explained to her that for a while, we needed to keep our contact secret.

I floated home. It had been completely overwhelming, and I suddenly realised that she had not been lost. She had always been there in my heart.

⟶⟨⟨⟩⟩⟵

The weeks went by, and slowly, we got to know each other. I told her that I did not expect to replace the mother who had raised her. In my mind, that was her real mother, the one who had nurtured and brought her up. I said that I was her birth mother but would be here for her now, if that was what she wanted. I went on to say that in different ways, she had two mothers.

I was so pleased that I could be here for her now because she was still young and needed a mum. She was divorced and had a family with two lovely young children of her own, and in time, another delightful child would be born. They are biologically my grandchildren. I can see family resemblances from her natural father's side and my own.

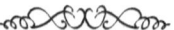

From my years of learning, I now have certain beliefs. While I realise others may not think like me, I know that there are those who do. I have read plenty of books from the minds of great thinkers, and I know for me what is true.

I believe that we choose the family that we want to be born into. I believe in reincarnation and that we come into each life with a set of lessons that we need to learn until we get it right and earn true eternal peace. I also believe as part of my learning, I was to give birth to this person and then give her to the people whom she had chosen to bring her up. This was the child they were meant to have.

As I said to her, *they* are her true family, and *mine* are an extension of that because of our biological connection. I have a special relationship with her because I am the one who brought her into the world. I am so grateful now that she chose me. I have in my life a beautiful young lady and her children, who have brought so much joy into my later years.

Most importantly, this reunion gave me final healing and peace after years of suffering, and now I understand.

I know that there are many different reasons and situations where outcomes like mine are not possible or simply don't happen. But for those who want to travel this path, I can only tell you that from my experience, *it has been completely worth it.*

It did take some time for my family to accept the new members, and it was stressful to say the least! My mother met "Mary" shortly before she died. My father didn't get that chance.

But we are all united in saying, "We are so happy to have you, Mary, in our lives."

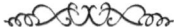

Before I finish this story, I will share with you a special moment. While it is one of many, it was particularly poignant.

Not long after meeting Mary, two tickets arrived in the mail. They were to a Christmas pantomime show in which she was the musical accompanist. I had by then confided in a close friend about our reunion, so I asked her along.

I wanted to blend into the audience because it was still overwhelming, and I felt rather nervous. After all, it was so new. But as soon as Mary saw me, she came rushing up, pleased that I was there.

The curtains rose, and there she was, seated at the piano. My heart skipped a beat as she began to play, and I was carried away to that place of eternal bliss. I felt justified in that moment as I realised how accomplished she was. I was thankful to her parents for providing the lessons that I could not give her and for raising her so well just as I had wanted. She is a beautiful person and a musical star. *Thank you, dear God, for making me whole again.*

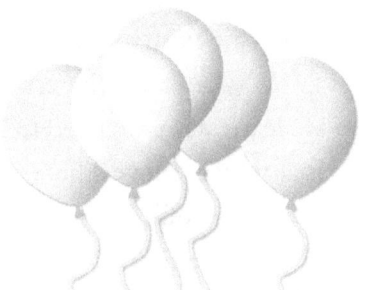

CHAPTER 15

And All Your Walls

O afflicted one, storm-tossed and not comforted,
behold, I will set your stones in antinomy,
and lay your foundations with sapphires.
I will make your pinnacles of agate,
and your gates of carbuncles,
and all your walls of precious stones.
—Isaiah 11-12

(October 2011)

This is only a small sample of that which is written. There is much more, but I think it sums up my journey and how life is for me now. I found passages like this in my Bible when I was desperately seeking answers. I highlighted the text and marked the pages. I read them over and over again. They comforted me and helped in giving me a strength that I never knew I had.

This verse still inspires me with a faith that tells me that all is attainable. We do not know when and where, but I trust that it will be given to us when we learn what we need to learn and live only from our heart, from that which is love. There, we find God, a state of being that we can all be part of.

Of course, for each of us, the timing is different, but we will all get there eventually. I have always been a deep thinker and pondered on the reason for life. After all the years of searching for answers, it is simple to me now. Love created us so that we would love too, but we have to learn how to love, and that may take many lifetimes.

I have been writing this story over the past two years. As I arrive at the last part, I see that it has been a journey within a journey. I wasn't aware of its true meaning until now. I knew that my life was evolving. My instincts told me that certain things were happening as I travelled through my grief, but I did not realise that I was learning so much along the way.

It is not only through losing my husband that I have grown. At the same time this was happening, I was also dealing with another loss. I wanted to include this story but decided then that the timing wasn't right. At present, it is of such a sensitive nature that I had to consider those involved, including my beloved brother, before I wrote! My brother has recently been diagnosed with frontal lobe dementia.

It first came to my attention that there was something seriously wrong with my brother for over two years ago just before Mike died. My brother changed from the person he had been, and it seemed to happen rather rapidly; however, in hindsight, it had started some time before. I feel like I have had a double loss in the last two years—my husband and a brother who is not the same person that he was previously.

It wasn't until lately that I realised that I was grieving the loss of that brother and addressed the sadness in me. I have accepted that my brother will not get better and his time here is limited. It has been extremely difficult to deal with, but I am clear in my mind now. While I still have feelings of sadness that this has happened to him, I understand that this is his journey.

One of the most important lessons that I have learned is that of compassion. I had always considered myself a compassionate person, but it wasn't real. Now that I have stopped feeling sorry for myself, I feel for others in a genuine way. I feel it from my heart and mind, and rather than let it overwhelm me, I can offer support in a positive way.

Where once I would try *to fix* everything and would consequently have high anxiety if I couldn't, I have surrendered and realised that I can't change another person's situation or take on their pain. It is not my right to do so. I can only offer comfort from that about which I have learned.

Acceptance is the key; however, accepting a situation that one cannot change takes time. When we surrender to it, we are set free. I have said that I had accepted Mike's passing, and that is true; however, it wasn't until the second anniversary that I fully let him go.

I also realised then that I had not grieved properly for the loss of my parents. I had no time because so much had been happening since then. And I was still caught up in sadness over my brother's illness.

In the month leading up to the anniversary, I had been experiencing a range of emotions, and I felt exhausted. That was when it all came to a head!

My daughters noticed that I was not myself and urged me to take some time off. I did this by getting more rest and slowly cleaning my house in the spring.

While I was doing this, I felt that I was uncluttering not only my house but my life as well. I decided that I wanted to stay in the home Mike and I had shared but that I wanted to make it mine now. I threw out a lot of things that reminded me of the past and arranged to have work done to bring new life to it.

I got rid of items from under the house. This was mainly the bits and pieces that Mike had collected and used. Afterwards, I could not believe what a difference it made, not only to the space below but inside the house as well. It had the effect of making *it* and also *myself* feel lighter.

I put a large statue of Buddha underneath my deck; Kaitlyn had given this to me as a gift the first Christmas after Mike' passing. I placed him in a spot that looked out to the garden. This added to the sense of peace that I was starting to feel now in and around my home.

While I was clearing out the things that I no longer wanted, I did much sorting through and reminiscing. I took time to remember my loved ones who had passed and carried out my own rituals. I lined up photos of my family for whom I hadn't fully grieved, including my brother.

I made an altar and burned white candles. I played the beautiful music of the "Gregorian Chant" sung by the Choir of the Monks of the Abbey of Santo Domingo de Silos. This music touched a chord in me that I felt directly in my heart. I wept and emptied the traces of lingering grief from the bowels of my being. After this, I did feel better. I felt more peaceful and calmer.

I planned to spend the day of the second anniversary quietly. I intended to watch one of Mike's favourite movies *Ghost*, have a takeaway dinner, and drink a glass of wine with a box of tissues handy. However, these plans didn't quite work out. It seemed that God had other ideas.

It was late afternoon when my phone rang. It was the sister of my friend and neighbour who had been admitted to hospital the night before. She gave me an update on her condition and asked if she could call in. I told her that would be fine. I had known her for some time but didn't see her often.

Mandy and I sat in the garden, and as we shared a glass of wine, we chatted away. I told her that it was the second anniversary of Mike's passing. She uttered words in sympathy and then went on to say that it would be five years the following day since she had lost her only daughter to cancer. I forgot about me at that moment and truly felt for this woman who had lost her beautiful daughter at just thirty-six.

Mandy had only come for a short visit, but we talked into the night. We shared wine. We shared a meal, and most importantly, we shared our grief. It was late when Mandy left, but we both expressed how beneficial this time had been.

Mandy was to tell me later that sharing in this way had helped her get through the days ahead and made the remembering a lot easier. It certainly helped me too, and I clearly saw that there were other people who had suffered like me and more.

I didn't get around to watching the movie *Ghost* until some weeks later, and when I did, it had a minimal effect on my emotions. It is said to be one of the best love stories ever written, but it is a rather old movie now. After my own experiences that were real, I thought it a little second-hand.

I have just realised that I haven't felt Mike on my shoulder for quite some time. Now that I have truly accepted his passing, I wonder if his spirit has gone. But no matter what, we will meet up again. I am not sure whether we will meet in my present lifetime or another.

I have been doing some research regarding reincarnation and soul mates. It has been truly enlightening and fits in with my own thoughts on this matter. And from what I read, it appears that the spirit of a loved one can stay around for weeks and sometimes months to see that their family is being cared for.

According to many learned people, the spirit then attains a higher vibration and moves on through other dimensions until it is out of contact with the ordinary humans on earth—except through someone who has the psychic ability to reach them.

I have also been wondering and gauging opinion on whether a departed soul or soul mate can choose to come back to a loved partner in a different body so that they can go on together unto eternity. I found some written thoughts on this. I had questioned whether the spirit could re-enter a body or only did this at a certain time before a baby was born. Or could it enter a body of any age?

There are articles written about this, and they say that yes, a spirit can re-enter another body at any age, given the right conditions.

Considering this information, I wondered about people who have personality changes. It is often said that he or she is a different person now, and maybe they are—

I found articles by the late psychic Ruth Montgomery and Marianne Williamson, articles that state two souls can agree to switch places. If the one in the body has gone as far as it can in its development and is ready to move on, it can leave and let the other spirit in. The new soul is usually a more evolved one and will serve in a different capacity. Apparently, a spirit can also "pop in" to a body to make contact with someone in this world.

They are referred to as "walk-ins," and according to the authors, this is happening more and more as we move toward the new age, specifically the age of Aquarius, or as it is commonly called the "Golden Age."

According to some predictions, the new age will begin in 2012. (There is even a date of December 21). This date is said to coincide with when the Mayan calendar finishes and when the world as we know it ends.

Many believe that this will be the time when Christ (the Second Coming) and other enlightened teachers like Buddha and Mohammed return. It is said that they may come back as walk-ins and lead us into the new age.

There are so many questions after we lose loved ones, and I recently experienced an encounter that had led me to wonder about "returning spirits."

I had gone to a local store to purchase some wine. It was shortly before the second anniversary of Mike's passing. I had gone there at times over the past two years, and I was usually caught up in my own thoughts as I wandered around considering the options.

This time, I had selected one bottle, and I was walking past two men talking when one of them turned around and looked straight at me. He said, "How are you?"

I did not know him, but there seemed to be something about him that was familiar. I replied, "I'm fine," and walked away.

I could hear his voice informing the other man, who was elderly, about different wines. I thought about how kind he sounded, and then he mentioned the wine that I had under my arm.

Normally, I would not have given this a second thought; however, there had been something different about this incident, and I could not forget the man's eyes when he had looked at me and asked how I was. There had been something about those eyes that I couldn't forget. It was like looking into the eyes of someone whom you have known for a long time.

In the following days, I could not get this person out of my mind, and this made me feel very emotional, especially as Mike's anniversary was approaching. I felt guilty because my focus was meant to be on my late husband, not another man. I had not considered or thought of anyone other than Mike, and I could not understand why this was happening now.

I decided to share this with a friend who had psychic abilities. She didn't seem surprised and said it was probably the spirit of Mike that I had seen in the stranger. She went on to say that he may have "popped in" to tell me that it was okay for me to move on and that it was time. She briefly described a man she saw in my future, and she said that he was a Christian.

I wondered if her predictions would happen in this dimension or another. *Maybe I already know him*, I thought.

As I mentioned before, when the process of spring-cleaning began, I made plans to have my house updated. It just seemed to happen with no real conscious effort on my part. It was as if the update was meant to be. I didn't want to change everything about the house but only blend some new things with what was already there.

I guess without fully realising it, I wanted to make the house mine. I wanted it to be simply lovely, not luxurious, but my oasis; somewhere I could feel peaceful and happy.

I called in tradesmen to do the work, and it all flowed smoothly. It seemed that they had been sent to me. Two painters came, and they worked on my house over several weeks. They were very helpful and went out of their way to make the renovation process easier.

One of them was a young man from Costa Rica. He was a gentle soul. Though he painted for a living, he was also a songwriter and musician. He told me that he had dreams of becoming famous. He brought me a demo tape of music featuring his band. It was made up of Latin, jazz, and reggae songs, and it sounded brilliant to me. I could tell that he was very talented.

I had a conversation with him one day, and I mentioned that I was going to give my house a name. I had been thinking of this recently, and I wanted to get a metal plaque made to put near my front door. I had been mulling over names with spiritual meaning, and I had come up with one.

I wanted my home to be called "The House of Light." There had been enough sadness. Now I wanted my house to be a place of peace and rest. I also wanted those who entered to feel that too. I asked the young man how the name was pronounced in Spanish.

He paused for a moment as if he was surprised. "That is a very good name," he said, and then he went on to say that it was *Casa de Luz*. I loved the sound of it in Spanish, and I told him so.

He went on to tell me that Luz was his mother's name, "Luz" meaning light. He then proceeded to say that his beloved mother had passed away some years before and that he had been devastated. He said that she had been a very good person, and in his words, she had been "close to God."

I could clearly see now that my life was evolving in a synchronistic way. There were many things occurring that were not mere coincidence. I could see a pattern emerging.

While I was bringing change to my house, I suddenly realised that I was introducing different cultural themes. I had done this in a subtle way, but it was there. I could see that this had occurred without me truly knowing.

I had blended the old and the new, and at the same time, I had adopted other places. I had gotten some pieces from my travels over the years, and lately while I had been renovating, I had sourced items locally. I now saw a theme that somehow had come together naturally.

I mentioned to the young painter that I seemed to have a mix of cultural bits and pieces. His words were that "all cultures are welcome in your house." And although I hadn't thought about it in that way before, I saw that this was true. I was telling my daughter Louise about this revelation, and she said, "Yes, Mum, you have always been accepting of other races and cultures."

I don't think that this has always been strictly correct. Before I had gotten to know people from different ethnic backgrounds and had exposure to them, I had been somewhat ignorant in my thinking. Because I had not been educated in this way, I was unaware, but I see now that we are truly all the same.

In the present time, there are those who are part of my family and who have come from other backgrounds, and I have grandchildren who are a mix of cultures. I love it this way, and I know it is meant to be.

Other meaningful "coincidences" occurred around the second anniversary of Mike's passing. Again, my intuition told me that they were not just normal happenings.

One morning, I awoke early and felt the urge to get up. I went outside into the garden. It was just after daybreak, and the birds were making their throaty calls as they gently stirred from rest. I sat on a seat, breathing in the soft smells of the new morning and enjoying the quiet, meditative moment.

My gaze wandered to the red rose bush that I had planted for Mike. It wasn't in flower yet, but my thoughts were on the small urn I had placed underneath it almost two years before.

Over the past week or so, I had been thinking about Mike's ashes, the little I had kept. I had wondered what part of his body they were from and decided that they were his heart. I had also made the decision to free them from the urn. I didn't know whether to scatter them at the spot where the rest had gone or to put them into the garden bed.

This morning, I knew that I was supposed to do it, and I silently asked Mike where he wanted them. A clear message came back:"With you … in the garden." I padded across the damp, dewy lawn in my slippers, and I unscrewed the lid on the little brass urn. I felt no sad emotion as I did this or as I tried to shake the ashes free. They would not budge, so I got some warm water and flushed them out and poured them around the red rose.

As soon as I released them into the soil, I felt a strong feeling of peace waft through my entire body, and my mind was blissfully still.

Thinking about this episode later, I came to the conclusion that by removing the ashes from the urn, I had taken the final step in setting Mike free, but then again, I decided that maybe it had been *him* setting *me* free.

On the day after the anniversary, I removed the engagement ring Mike had given me from my finger. This again had a liberating effect on me. I placed a pearl ring of my own on the second finger of my right hand. I felt then that I had reclaimed myself.

I had received an invitation to a Baptism. It had been an unexpected but pleasant surprise. It was to be held the week after the anniversary. I hadn't been to church for a long time, and I was looking forward to the occasion and the after-party. I knew it would be a big day as one side of the family was Italian.

I had bought a new dress, and on the day before the event, I had my hair done. I was leaving the hair salon when I saw a gorgeous flowering plant sitting outside the florist shop next door. I was transfixed. It was so beautiful.

I walked over and stood there for some time, looking at its lovely trumpeted white blooms. It had a tag attached that said it was a hippeastrum. I had heard of them but had not seen one, and it was a fine specimen. Also written on the tag was the name "the wedding dance." I felt the peaceful feeling (that was so familiar to me now) sweep through me, and I knew that I had to buy this lovely plant.

I took it home and put it on my deck near a window where I could see it from my living room. I kept looking at its beauty and wondered what its significance was in a spiritual sense.

I felt that it had something to do with the "wedding of souls," and I thought back to that time some years before, after my first spiritual experience when the spirit of Mike had called to mine and I had joined him again.

I went to the Baptism, which was held at a local Catholic church, and as I entered the building, I felt that I was in a state of bliss. The baby boy being baptised was adorable, and as family members said, "He was special." You could see it in his eyes. He had been here before.

In a way, I felt like I was also being baptised again into a new life. I had completely negated the past and was free to move on in peace and joy.

After a day of happiness and celebration, I returned home, and that night, I had a "dream." I can only describe it in a physical sense. The strength of the "dream" woke me up. I felt the experience through my entire body, and for a moment, it scared me.

But it wasn't a dream. It was real, and what I felt was an energy surging through me. For an instant, I thought it might have been the spirit of Mike (as I had felt that first Christmas after I had lost him), but then my instincts told me it wasn't him. I wondered if another spirit had "possessed" my body. (Possession is when a spirit from the "lower realms" inhabits a body uninvited.) This really freaked me out.

Suddenly, the surging within me stopped, and I felt calm. It came to me then that it was my true spirit entering into me. I guessed that after all that I had been through, I had come home to myself, my real self, my Christ self.

It has taken me some time to fully comprehend this, but now that I do, I am walking a new path—in body and soul.

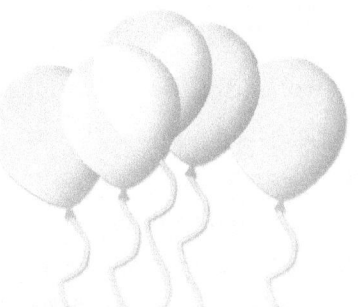

CHAPTER 16

Reflections

I wrote this section six months later. (May 2012.)

Presently, I feel that I am caught between two worlds. I have progressed so far along the track and have been constantly learning. I have been high, and I have been low. This has not gone unnoticed by those around me, and I don't expect them to understand because I only *just* understand it myself. Of course, I have been through a period of grief that would account for much of this, but alongside this process, I have also been awakening to the nature of real life, the one that we are meant to have.

As I have said from the beginning of my story, it has been a journey of spiritual learning as well as an emotional and physical one. It started on my fiftieth birthday, and now I feel it is coming to a climax. Throughout this journey, I have reached the state of higher consciousness and felt the bliss of it. But I did not stay there and could not stay there. Ultimately, I would come back to the reality of the world and more "obstacles" in my way.

I found this very difficult. I wanted to stay in that place where everything was so wonderful. I felt completely peaceful there, and I looked on my life from a mind that saw only beauty. What seemed important or urgent had no meaning, and there was no time attached. I felt connected to all around me and deeply content in just being. I felt joy there and looked on life in a completely positive way. I felt complete, and I could clearly see all my needs being met.

Now, more and more, I feel the peace of that higher world. (I know the timing is right now.) I feel myself becoming separated from the lower world. It frustrates and saddens me because of the negativity that is part of it.

It is like I am living in two worlds.

From what I am learning and believe, we are in the time of "ascension." We are ascending to a higher dimension. We are leaving the third dimension and proceeding to the fifth, which will be heaven on earth.

It is said that there are vibrational effects being felt within the physical body and within the earth itself. (There is information written in books and online about this.) And increasingly, I am feeling change in myself. It seems that I am tuning into a different *frequency!*

I believe that a new age and a new world are imminent. I feel the energy and excitement of it in my being. It is like anticipating an exotic destination during a long period of travel, but I also know that this place will be the most magnificent of all.

I don't know why I see and feel this, but I am truly blessed to be among those who do. I am certainly not alone in my views. I have met others who share my thinking. And there are many people throughout the world who know as much as me, and some even know a lot more.

It is said that we are forming a circle around the earth. I believe this thinking has been coming through to us from the spirit world because we are receptive to it. And through sharing what we know of a *new reality*, we can assist others by taking them into the light with us. Then together, *we can* create paradise.

Apparently, this thinking is filtering through more rapidly now, and more people are becoming enlightened. I believe that the healing of the world can only happen by divine intervention.

I know that my search for true and lasting peace will be over soon; the time for it is almost here. As it is said in *A Course in Miracles*, "God will take the final step."

And as for Mike, he *is* still around. Our spirits are united. In whatever form, we *will* be together again, and this time, we will be in perfect harmony because we have both learned that which we needed to learn . . . and now we know.

Endnote

This story goes on, and I could keep on writing; however, for now these are my final words. You can ask questions on my website—www.loss-grief-innerpeace.com *There you will also find links to my BlogSpot and Facebook page.

The book that I left for Harley in the Volunteer office at the hospital has been found! Harley made inquiries, and now two and a half years later, he has returned *A Course in Miracles* to me.

He visited today and said that he has looked through it but feels that he does not have time presently to commit to the "course."

All things happen for good reason, and maybe he was not meant to do it. We are all on our own paths! But the book has played a part in my journey. Hmm—I don't think that it is merely a coincidence that it has turned up now. Its timing is precise, as it coincides with me finishing this story!

And I can see that through meeting Harley and sharing my thoughts with him, a connection was made. This is what I would call a miracle, wouldn't you? I would like to sincerely thank Harley for his assistance in editing my story.

He is one of many angels here and above who have appeared to guide and assist me through this process of self-discovery and writing this book. I haven't done it alone. Thank you all!

NB: Liz and I were talking today about a return visit to Mana in July. (It is now May.). She told me how excited she is and that she can't wait to go. She then went on to say, "I suppose the time there will pass too quickly!"

I said, "It will be perfect, and we will make the most of every moment."

And Liz replied with a statement that was also a question: "Yes, but we won't go again, will we?"

My answer to her was this: "Probably not, but we will go to other places." My feeling is that we won't need to, because paradise will be wherever we are!